MW01056009

"Nurses are natural storytellers and Brittney demystify blogging concepts and make it easy for nurses to feel confident to start a blog or expand their current online influence. This book is thorough, fun, and motivating. It's a must-read for any nurse who wants to leave a lasting legacy in nursing and life."

Donna Cardillo, RN, MA, CSP
The Inspiration Nurse and author of *Falling Together: How to Find Balance, Joy, and Meaningful Change When Your Life Seems to be Falling Apart*

"Brittney Wilson, The Nerdy Nurse and Kati Kleber, Fresh RN, are considered two of the top resources and thought leaders in social media with deep expertise in blogging. Nurses Guide to Blogging is a value-packed book where Brittney and Kati generously share insider secrets and the actual tactics on a developing a true business and brand. Get out your highlighter; this book is a keeper!"

Michelle Podlesni
President - National Nurses in Business Association
Author of *Unconventional Nurse® Going from Burnout to Bliss!*

"The perfect package. What I love best about this book is that it is REAL. While Brittney and Kati know their stuff and have TONS of resources for the new nurse blogger- the real world examples, stories from personal experiences, and lessons learned are what makes this book a fantastic read. After reading this book, you will not just be another nurse blogger. Using the tools in this text will put you on the path to blogging success in a sustainable career!"

Elizabeth Scala, MSN/MBA, RN
Author of Bestselling Nursing from Within

THE NURSE'S GUIDE TO BLOGGING:

Building a Brand and a Profitable Business as a Nurse Influencer

Also by Brittney Wilson, BSN RN

The Nerdy Nurse's Guide to Technology (Sigma Theta Tau International)

Also by Kati Kleber, BSN RN CCRN

The Anatomy of a Super Nurse: The Ultimate Guide to Becoming Nursey (American Nurses Association)

Admit One: What You Must Know When Going to the Hospital But No One Actually Tells You (American Nurses Association)

What's Next? The Smart Nurse's Guide to Your Dream Job (American Nurses Association)

THE NURSE'S
GUIDE TO BLOGGING

Building a Brand and a
Profitable Business as a Nurse
Influencer

By Brittney Wilson, BSN RN
and
Kati Kleber, BSN RN CCRN

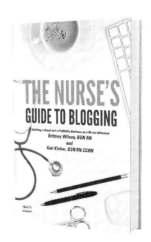

HealthMediaAcademy.com

Health Media Academy Publishing

www.healthmediaacademy.com

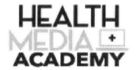

*To nurses past and present who have labored
to move our profession forward.*

About the
Authors

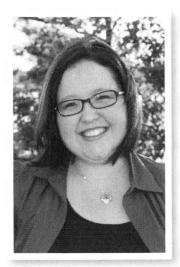

Brittney Wilson, BSN RN is the nurse behind TheNerdyNurse.com. She is an award-winning author and blogger, international keynote speaker, and influencer in the nursing and healthcare IT communities.

Established in 2010, The Nerdy Nurse® is a leading nursing and technology blog that is consistently listed as one of the top nursing blogs on the web. In fact, out of the 20 most popular nursing sites online, The Nerdy Nurse is the only site fully owned and operated by a Registered Nurse.

Kati Kleber, BSN RN CCRN is the nurse behind FreshRN.com. She has experience in cardiac stepdown as well as neuroscience critical care. A veteran author, blogger, podcaster, and speaker on top nursing trends, Kati has been recognized by Charlotte Business Journal as *2015 Nurse of the Year* and is a recipient of the *Great 100 Nurses of North Carolina* award. Kati has also been a featured source across a number of media outlets, including CNN, The Dr. Oz Show, U.S. News & World Report, The TODAY show, and many more.

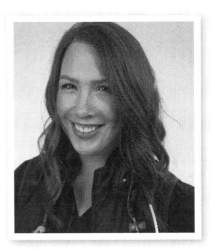

Ch. 1

3,344
× 10
―――――
0 0 0 0
3,3 4 0
3,3
―――――
33,440
words

1 6
418
× 8
――――――
33 4 4 = Ch. 1

Greg Vayrochuk
Jub, Jub Jub 8u
wor

418 words
418 pgs pr pgs.
418 x 8 = Intro

Contents

418x3

418 x 8

418x8

Chapter 5

Getting the Most
Out of This Book

This book was written from the perspective of Kati Kleber and Brittney Wilson. While we agree on most aspects of this ever-important (and evolving) topic, there are some times in which we have different perspectives or will provide our unique experience. The collective voice throughout the text is from both of us, and for ease of reading have utilized the pronoun "we". However, if one of us describes our personal experience or thought, we will indicate who is speaking within that respective section.

Furthermore, this book contains a large amount of information. This is not a book you can read, set down, and implement everything at once. As we will discuss, the process of building a platform takes time and is full of trial and error. Developing a successful platform is not a cookie-cutter, identical path. Like our patients, business is dynamic. Platforms evolve, new ones are introduced, and algorithms change. Additionally, different influencers have different passions and focuses and therefore what is an essential social media platform or marketing strategy for one may not be as crucial to another. Please keep that in mind.

To prevent yourself from feeling totally overwhelmed by a to-do list longer than a crashing patient admission, please follow these tips:

1. Read the book cover-to-cover before implementing any changes

2. Highlight like you did in nursing school (so, everything… right?)

3. As you read, take notes on things you'd like to implement, changes you'd like to make, things that have inspired you, and any ideas

4. Identify things that you need to do soon, later, and someday (short term, medium, and long term goals)

5. Think about an accountability partner you can share your goals with, get input, and check in with

Additionally, we mention many different terms, websites, programs, applications, and more. We often use the terms blog and website interchangeably. Throughout the book, you'll find textboxes in which we have defined common blogging terms, with a summary of definitions in one of the appendices in the back. Because blogging is ever changing, we've created a master list of links to everything we recommend at HealthMediaAcademy.com/ Resources. This will ensure you get to exactly the page you need, whether you're reading this in paperback or ebook. It will also allow us to make updates with new resources that may be more up to date than the text. And, in true nurse blogger form many of the links are affiliate links. By the end of this book, you'll learn how to do the same.

Alright! Let's get started, nurses!

Introduction

The online world is crowded.
There are millions, if not billions, of websites, social media accounts, blogs, podcasts, and videos online.

Standing out in a crowded sea of blogs and internet personalities is no small feat. Fortunately for you, being a nurse gives you a bit of an edge. You have an incredible arsenal of nursing skills that make you uniquely suited for both blogging and business. You're a planner, an organizer, prioritizer, and a great storyteller. But most importantly, you care about people.

The skills you use at the bedside, or even beyond, can help you become a profitable blogger or use a blog to grow a new or existing business. But, it's going to take hard work.

Just like the work of nursing is like an iceberg, so is blogging. What you see on the surface is nothing compared to what is hidden below the water or behind the scenes. Deciding to blog professionally is a great decision, but if you plan to get real results in terms of career advancement or income, it will require that you learn the tools of the trade and become comfortable using new technologies and skills. Of course, nurses do this every day, so you're already ahead of the game.

While readers may not realize how much work goes on behind the scenes, their tastes and needs are constantly evolving. You must be willing to grow and adapt with your audience as you both evolve. To run a successful business and blog you'll never stop learning.

Social media platforms are getting smarter. They know that people won't stay and hang out on their platform if it's not interesting to them. Therefore, they create algorithms to prioritize things they think the consumer will enjoy in their timelines, newsfeeds, or suggested sections. If you've ever wondered why pages you like on Facebook never seem to show up in your feed, these algorithms are to blame.

To top it off, people are distracted easily. If your content is not powerful and concise, people stop reading and move on. However, if they find your content valuable they'll stick around. They may even opt-in to your email list or share it on their social sites, exposing your content to many more people. As content creators, we have much to lose and much to gain. Every piece of content you put out into the world is a chance to win or lose. You want to find things that work and replicate. When things don't work, you will need to pivot. Knowing when to pivot and when to stay the course is critical. We'll help you learn how determine when that is.

Finally, there any many blogs and influencers providing similar information. So if one blog is generally valuable, but has polarizing or offensive content... people will just ignore, unfollow, unsubscribe, and go elsewhere. This is especially important to consider when you are blogging as a professional nurse. Nurses are naturally held to a higher standard. Blogging is no exception.

People are able to customize their online experience to what they find valuable, entertaining, and cool, and cut out the rest. While as a consumer, this is a wonderful thing... as a content creator, it forces you to step your game up tremendously. You have to raise the standards of your content and your brand to meet the needs of your ideal audience.

To compare this to the nursing world, it's kind of like core measures (we know, we're sorry!). Core measures are basically a standard of care the hospital must meet to receive Medicare and Medicaid reimbursement, with the ultimate goal of improving care and reducing cost. We don't know of many hospitals that can survive without reimbursement from Medicare and Medicaid, so this is a big deal. If the hospital isn't discharging their heart failure patients with appropriate education, or administering beta blockers after surgery if they were received prior, or if blood cultures were not obtained within 24 hours of admission and prior to the initiation of antibiotics for pneumonia patients, the hospital isn't getting reimbursed. As a patient, this can be a wonderful thing. As a hospital, this creates a challenge. It also creates negative cash flow if they are not compliant with best practices. Because a hospital's bank account will suffer if they do not meet the standards of core measures, they are forced to comply.

At the end of the day, it's better for everyone if we're encouraging better patient outcomes. Similarly, it's better for everyone if we're finding quality content easily online, without being distracted by things that are low quality, not valuable, or not appropriate for that specific consumer.

A Marathon, Not a Sprint

The process of growing a blog and a brand can be compared to caring for stroke patients. Stroke recovery is quite a long process, as it frequently requires months for the brain to heal. Everyone's brain will heal differently also, so it can be difficult to talk about a prognosis with patients and families, especially early on.

 Creating an engaged community who cares so much about what you have to say that they'll share it with their peer group takes time. Building trust doesn't happen overnight.

Shortcuts are fruitless endeavors. While you could go buy followers on various social media platforms, they will not be engaged or actually care about who you are or what you are doing.

Readers shouldn't be thought of as merely a means to a financial end. If your goal is to blog purely for income, you're doing it wrong. Sure you could create and sell an info-product that is mildly helpful and maybe make a little money in the short term, but that won't last long.

You also don't want to exploit yourself or your profession. Being a professional nurse on social means you're held to higher standards and your actions will be viewed more critically than the public at large. When it comes to posting scandalous or inappropriate content in an attempt to gain followers or traffic, just don't. While we're in a world where sex sells, do you really want to leverage your professional platform by posting compromising pictures of yourself to gain a higher follower count?

These shortcuts will only get you so far. It's kind of like when you have a septic patient with a really high fever; while you can give them some Tylenol to help with the fever, what they really need are some IV antibiotics. Your Tylenol may fix the fever, but the underlying issue must be addressed.

Creating a successful and valuable platform with engaged followers is a long process. It takes quite a bit of time for it to become financially rewarding. You must sow value into your community before you can reap the benefits. "

When Sowing Turns Into Reaping

One of the leaders in the entrepreneur communities is Gary Vaynerchuk (Garyvee for short). He's written quite a few great books on this topic, but one of my favorites is *Jab, Jab, Jab, Right Hook: How to Tell Your Story in a Noisy Social World*[1]. While this book was written in 2013 (which seems like a lifetime in this constantly evolving world of social media), it has some key principles that are essential to understand as you're developing your brand and platform.

We are not going to go into all of the details, as we highly recommend reading it cover-to-cover, but we do want to point out one of the important concept he outlines: micromarketing. The title of the book is *Jab, Jab, Jab, Right Hook*; but another way of saying that is Give, Give, Give, Ask. You will be providing valuable, unique content to your community over and over again, and then finally ask them to do something.

For most bloggers, the income isn't instant. It can take many months or years to build a following substantial enough to monetize. It can be done sooner, but you really have to hustle to provide enough value to not be perceived as a cash grab.

How Kati Got Started

I was working on my blog for a year before creating a product. I provided a year of free, valuable, and reliable content to new nurses, and then finally independently published a book after building a little hype and behind the scenes action around it. I priced my book low ($12.99 for print, $7.99 for electronic), as to make it affordable for most, sold it on Amazon, and sold more than 18K copies in three years. I have since landed a publishing deal with the American Nurses Association for two additional titles, and a second edition of the first.

---

1 Vaynerchuk, Gary. *Jab, Jab, Jab, Right Hook: How to Tell Your Story in a Noisy, Social World*. First edition. HarperBusiness, 2013.

How Brittney Got Started

In 2008, I became a nurse. To describe my first year as turbulent would be an understatement. Because of the challenges I endured, I started a blog in 2010 to share resources and recommendations for dealing with bullying and other issues encountered as a new nurse. I poured time, energy, and effort into my blog for more than three years before I earned any money from it. In fact, I had to get over the guilt associated with earning income from something I felt could be only altruistic in nature. However, the offers to sponsor content came continuously. I ultimately made peace with the fact that I could create content to help nurses and also earn an income source. Years of free content and resources were available before I earned one red cent. Once I was ready to monetize, the opportunities were almost limitless allowing The Nerdy Nurse to evolve to one of the most popular nursing blogs on the web. During this journey, I've had the pleasure of traveling internationally as a professional speaker, writing the award-winning book *The Nerdy Nurse's Guide to Technology*, and continuing to help nurses while I grow my business.

Nurses and Entrepreneurs Must Always Think Big Picture

What we're basically trying to make clear is success and financial rewards from blogging do not happen overnight. At the end of the day, your bottom line must be your passion, not your wallet. It takes giving a lot of yourself over time, by investing into the best interests of your community every day, with a big-picture mentality.

This is just like nurses implement their care plans every shift. While the patient doesn't want to ambulate because they're in pain today, the nurse knows they must motivate and encourage their patient to walk because they have an understanding of the big picture: not walking today will make it harder tomorrow, and will ultimately delay discharge and healing.

Constantly focusing on the big picture will help you to determine how valuable a potential project or strategy is. You can think back to it and see if it helps to facilitate your passion and aligns with the big picture, or if it distracts from it.

As a nurse, you already have great problem-solving and planning skills to help you be successful as a nurse blogger and in any nursing business. Remember all those care plans you wrote in nursing school? How about all that assessing, planning, and intervening you do on a daily basis? You can leverage the same skills you use to plan and provide excellent patient care to plan for your success as a nurse entrepreneur.

We encourage you to create your nurse entrepreneur care plan.

- What is the problem you've identified?
- How do did you know it was a problem (assessment data)?
- What's your plan to address this problem?
- What are your interventions?
- And how is it going implementing them (evaluation)?

Let's take Kati's brand and mission and create a care plan.

Assessment
- Nurse Burnout Statistics
- Personal experience of nurse burnout
- Do not have initiatives for nurse burnout
- Burnout myths & stigma
- Wellness Retreats & Workshops

Diagnosis - Knowledge deficit in nurse expert burnout r/t lack of knowledge, resources and support AEB nurses trying but & going to problem.

Assessment	• Personal experience of being unprepared after graduation • High new grad turnover rates • Many new nurses requiring additional support and guidance • Need for residency programs • Many new grads on social media supporting one another
Nursing Diagnosis	• Unprepared new graduate nurse population r/t lack of practical knowledge, skills and support to be successful at the bedside AEB high new graduate nurse turnover rates, new nurses leaving the profession, and personal experience
Planning	• Create a blog and social platforms to support new nurses *exp knot* • Write a concise handbook • Record a podcast • Record a weekly video series • Speak at nursing schools • Partner with nursing-related companies
Implementation	• Blog successfully created and updated to full website of resources • 5 books written • 1 podcast with seasons created • 4 weekly videos created • Spoken at 4 nursing schools • Multiple contracts with various nursing-related companies
Evaluation	• Fine-tuning content creation for blog to meet the needs of students • Need to devote more time to create blog posts • Books written, 25K+ copies sold total, need to create supplemental material • Podcast created with over 30K downloads, compiling notes • Only 4 videos created – more time needed to plan, create, reference, publish – will reattempt • Must ensure to evaluate if interested companies align with my bottom line and nursing diagnosis

Use your care plan, or in this case, your nurse blog business plan to constantly evaluate the success of your blog.

Continually sow into your community with meaningful and valuable content, rooted in your passion. Be willing to pivot when things aren't working. Listen to your audience and connect with them in a meaningful way. Ultimately, you will begin to reap the benefits of an engaged and passionate community.

That is how you turn clicks into conversions, casual visitors into brand advocates, and online acquaintances into professional partnerships.

So, Who is Your Community?

We assume if you want to start a blog about something, that means you are passionate about something. We also assume that by creating a blog, you're hoping to share what you're passionate about with others, or that you're hoping to fill a void in the marketplace with this passion. As you're creating content and getting people to care about it, you're creating a community.

This community is comprised of people who merely come and consume your content and leave, others who consume your content and share with others, and finally people who consume your content, share with others, and act as an advocate for you.

The identity of this community is your brand.

When people go to Twitter, Facebook, or Instagram and want to see if you're sharing your content there as well, they'll look for your brand. They'll follow, like, subscribe, and maybe even reblog your content. They'll interact with people who also enjoy your brand in comment sections, through tweets, and live videos.

Think of your audience and community as your patient. Only this nurse-to-patient relationship will hopefully never end.

How does that relationship begin? You introduce yourself, tell them the plan and what you're going to do for them today. You build trust. You build rapport. You get to know them and understand what's important to them. You meet their support system. You speak to their needs. You show up when you say you will. You try to be motivating when they need motivation. You try to be comforting when they need to be comforted. You solve problems for them. You read situations, anticipate needs and obstacles, you know when to change your approach, and empathize at every step along the way.

Just like the nurse is the leader and advocate of the patient's care team, you are the leader and advocate for your community.

CHAPTER 1

THE POWER AND POTENTIAL OF
THE NURSE BLOGGER

"How very little can be done under the spirit of fear."

- Florence Nightingale

"Everyone can tell you the risk. An entrepreneur can see the reward."

– Robert Kiyosaki

The registered nurse is a very educated, informed, and trusted person who reaches one patient at a time.
The blogger is an innovative, passionate, thought-provoking person who has the potential to reach the masses.

Leverage these two roles appropriately, and the sky's the limit.

The Potential for Personal Growth

If you picture yourself standing on a stage, delivering your message and passion to the crowd; your blog is the stage that is holding you up, and social media is the spotlight. In this book, we will discuss how to build a strong stage and a big spotlight. Both of these aspects are essential to getting your voice heard; however, we cannot create the message for you. You must know what you want to say. There must be a fire within you that you yearn to share with your audience. This book will give you the tools to build your stage and turn on the spotlight, but it's up to you to stand on the stage and deliver a powerful and valuable message to the world.

A blog is a great stage for you to get your message across for many reasons. First, it's affordable. With minimal financial investment (less than $100 in most cases), you can create an attractive website to showcase what you have to offer. People can go to your website, and learn about you and your passion with just a few clicks. There are so many resources and tools available to make this process as streamlined as it could possibly be. With so many resources out there it can get confusing, so we are going to take all of those different floating pieces in the online world and pull them together for the nurse who wants to build a successful blog.

Next, a blog is easily updated. With working 12-hour shifts, taking call, and being present for the rest of your life, it's hard to find a lot of time to devote to maintaining a blog. The wonderful thing about blogs is, once you have it set up how you would like it, the process of adding new content is quick and streamlined. Every time you want to add more content, you don't have to make a PowerPoint, or design the entire page each time, you merely add your new content. The hard work is done, and you can focus on what is most valuable: creating content.

Finally, blogs are highly customizable. You can make it unique to you. There is no perfect format or way it must look to be successful. As the blogger and owner, this is your space and your passion; put your spin on it. There isn't a corporate template you must follow.

If leveraged appropriately, you can do something that wasn't possible 15 years ago: you can communicate your passion directly to your target audience all across the globe, and earn income at the same time. How amazing is that? Talk about job satisfaction!

While it may take years to be able to live off of the income earned from your online endeavors, the potential is there. How quickly you get there depends on multiple factors with the primary variable being you.

The Potential for Professional Growth

Blogging is a great endeavor for many people with various professional backgrounds, but the potential for the nurse is particularly valuable.

The nursing professional stands much to gain with educated nurses writing blogs and being behind successful social media platforms. We can inform and educate patients; empower, educate and encourage one another; and we can network and collaborate with other nurses and healthcare team members all around the world, instantly.

Maybe the nurses over at Johns Hopkins completed a research study about their new fall prevention program that's proven to be highly successful, or maybe the nurses down at Duke instituted a new effective clinical ladder program that the staff is really excited about, or maybe Michael Ackerman, DNS, RN, APRN-BC, CENP, FCCM, FAANP (nationally recognized speaker on sepsis) tweeted some new information about sepsis. This is all highly valuable information worthy of being shared and utilized by many nurses, worldwide.

Blogging and social media makes professional collaboration instant and free. You no longer have to wait for a yearly conference to get a sneak peek into what other institutions are doing across the country. You can connect with these hospital, schools, nursing leaders, bedside nurses, and educators instantly through social media. Harnessed appropriately, the potential impact of conscientious nurses leveraging blogs and social media on nursing research, patient satisfaction, patient safety, peer support, and growth is profound.

Furthermore, if you clearly define your niche and have specific experience to strengthen your credibility, you have the opportunity to become an expert in your area.

13

CHAPTER 2

DEFINING YOUR
MESSAGE AND NICHE

S o now that we have talked about the profound potential benefits of nurse bloggers and social media influencers, let's dive deeper into what drives your website, platforms, and content.

Before buying a domain name, securing social media handles, and writing blog posts, it is absolutely critical to define your passion and purpose as specifically as possible. This will help you to define your niche and be the foundation for your brand.

The Problem You're Solving

"I want to help nurses," is a really broad topic in a saturated market. Try to be as specific as possible. You need to know who you want to help and what you want to help them with. Essentially, you want to be able to say "I help _____ with _____ by doing _____."

Consider these questions:

- Is your passion making it easier for nurses to find jobs?
- Is it your passion to address the major disconnect between human resources and onboarding nurses?
- Do you want to support nurses who experience of bullying?

- Do you want to help nurses who are struggling with nurse-life balance?
- Do you want to help nurses live a healthier lifestyle?
- Do you want to help patients navigating the healthcare process?

You're likely passionate about many things so this is really just a matter of narrowing it down. Ask yourself a few questions:

- What do I know that I can teach other nurses?
- What could I write about for years without getting bored?
- What do I see nurses or patients struggle with that I can help to address?
- What is something I struggle with that I can learn about and teach others as I learn at the same time?

Finally, do some research to find out if the problem you want to address is actually a problem for a given audience. Join some Facebook grounds and ask questions about that subject. See how many people respond. Do this a few times and see whether or not people are interested in talking about the topic or have struggled with the topic. You don't want to build an entire brand and business based around a solution for a problem that doesn't exist.

Whatever you decide is your niche, ask yourself: could you write blog post after blog post, find resources, and engaged in meaningful conversation around this topic for years to come? Would you be okay doing that and not making any money for a while? Eventually, is there a product I could create that aligns with this topic?

Your Message Will Evolve

What you decide today is not set in stone. Even if you perform a ton of research and nail a real problem, your idea could come at the wrong time. In business, there are often times when you have to pivot. Sometimes this means narrowing your focus other times this means choosing and entirely new niche altogether. Before making the decision to pivot weigh the pros and cons and ensure the decision you're making has strategic advantages in the long run rather than feeling right in the moment.

Our brands and messages have evolved over many years of blogging. As we've refined our niche and focus, we've seen our traffic and income increase. We didn't start out as experts and are always learning something new. You've heard the phrase "A nurse that knows everything is a dangerous nurse." The same holds true for blogging.

We both spent considerable time working full time as nurses while growing our brands. This meant answering emails after 12-hour shifts, writing blog posts for other sites for free just to get our name out there, and cold calling various prominent nursing websites to see if we could be featured.

What's Your Bottom Line?

Clearly define your passion. Why are you blogging to begin with? What are your goals? What must happen, even if people disagree with you or are negative, or if you spent money in the wrong place, or if you didn't make a dime? Ultimately, what is your bottom line?

For example, Kati's bottom line is growing and supporting new nurses. Jon Haws over at NRSNG.com, his bottom line is providing "ah-ha" moments to nursing students, Brittney's bottom line is improving the lives of nurses and the patients they serve through the use of technology.

Identifying your bottom line will not only help you define your niche, but when you find yourself trying to figure out your next priority, or when you're not sure if an opportunity is a good fit, you'll be able to come back to it to aid in your decision. Staying focused on your bottom line at each step will streamline processes, prevent wasted time and energy, and maintain your high level of personal and professional job satisfaction as you progress.

Nichelle things Bottom line is
pretty nurse knot,

An Important Aspect of Kati's Bottom Line

Faith is something that guides how I live my life, and my blog is no exception. When I'm stuck, not sure about my next priority, or if I'm not sure if what I'm currently doing really aligns with who I am and my purpose, then it's a definitely a signal to me that I need to step back, and step into prayer. Attempting to stay centered in this helps me to have perspective and step outside of myself and think of my audience as a whole, and how I can best serve them. It has been a very reliable and consistent indicator for me.

If I feel a check in my spirit, or if thinking about an opportunity gives me anxiety and not peace, I know that I need to pause. It's also been something I lean into when I'm not sure about something I have posted, if I later decide I handled something poorly online, or discover I provided inaccurate information. Audiences appreciate when you can humble yourself and say you've screwed up. Publically admitting to being a fallible human makes you *more* authentic to your audience, and people end up trusting you more because they know you'll admit when you're wrong. My faith has been and will continue to be part of my bottom line.

Clearly Define Your Niche

Now that you know your bottom line and have identified your passion; you need to define you your niche. Ask yourself: who is your audience? What specific content will you be focusing on? It is a precise nursing specialty or a group of problems you see in the profession? Be as specific as possible. The more you can define and narrow this audience and define your niche, the faster you can become a leader in this area.

Niche: A small specialized topic or focus that appeals to a subset of the population.

For example, mom bloggers are a highly-saturated market. There are hundreds of thousands of mom bloggers. To get to the top of this market and become a leader it would take years of very fine-tuned, specific efforts, lots of luck, and most likely a financial investment. However, if you're a mom blogger who has a passion for different kinds of olive oils, and enjoys sampling kinds from different regions and creating kid-friendly recipes with oil profiles – that would be a different story. It would be much easier to become known as an olive oil expert than it would to be on parenting.

Nursing is a huge field. With 3.8 million and counting in the US, writing a blog for the entire profession is going to take quite a bit of calculated efforts, substantial networking, and incredible skill to get to be known as an authority. If you narrowed your niche from the entire profession, to say… transplant recovery room nurses; your chances of success are much higher. Instead of writing general articles that the major nursing website and blogs have already covered, you could write content about the specific struggles of working in such a specific and intense environment. You can give feedback and advice to those already in the specialty or interested in making transition. You can become the top online influencer in transplant nursing.

The more specific you can get about your audience, and the more focused you can get with creating content solving problems of that niche, the more valuable your content becomes.

This is how you become known. This is how people find you. This is how you make an impact within your passion. It doesn't matter if you're an expert in that area today. Building a blog will force you to learn and eventually become as skilled as anyone in that area. To be truly successful, you must specialize your content around a niche and ensure all your content relates to it. You cannot just put content out there and hope someone finds it. That is like throwing a diamond ring in the middle of ocean and hoping someone knows to look for it there without providing a map.

The nursing profession is like the Pacific Ocean. Narrow your niche down to the Gulf of California, then down to Lake Mead, then down to a swimming pool. It's a heck of a lot easier to find a diamond ring in something the size of a swimming pool than an ocean. It's small enough that they won't need a map.

Your Online Presence

Next, decide what you want your online presence to look like. You already know your bottom line, your passion, and your niche. How can you wrap that in a tight little package so others know what you're all about? This is what needs to occur so you can define your brand.

What do you want your brand to be about? Your personality should shine through your writing, community, images, and engagement. Do you enjoy the outdoors? Are you a traveler? Are you a reader? Do you love TV? Do you nerd out whenever a new Apple product comes out? Are you a diehard football fan?

People love to see the personality of the blogger to shine through into their work. You're not a faceless company. You're a nurse with a unique personality and it should be evident in what you do online. People are more likely to engage online when they know they're talking to a real person and not a faceless company. This is how you begin to build an authentic community around your brand. People want to know about you; not just the professional side, but all of who you are as a person. It is much easier to relate to someone and trust them if you know more about them outside of what they do for a living.

Nurses actually have leg up when building a brand. We're consistently voted as the most trustworthy profession, so the public has a natural inclination to trust us. Being a nurse is sort of like being in special club (and potentially, the coolest club). Nurses also relate to other nurses.

Marketing has changed rapidly; arguably as rapidly as the healthcare industry that we live and breathe every shift! In the past, people had a business side of life and a personal side of life. With social media, people love having glimpses into people's personal lives. Your brand should substantiate your passion, personality and purpose. People don't just want to know what you do, they want to know who you are. So, if you're a nurse whose platform is centered on wellness like Kelsey over at thewellnesschicks.com, people would love a photo of your shopping cart, or how you prepare your meals for your shifts, or your favorite brand of coconut oil.

In the past, you'd only see celebrities endorsing products to increase a company's credibility. "Man, if Beyoncé is in a Pepsi commercial, she must really like Pepsi," is what the consumer mindset used to be. Times have changed, and the consumer is smarter. People know Beyoncé doesn't stay in the shape she's in by drinking Pepsi, Shaq doesn't really drive a Dodge around, and Kim Kardashian isn't wearing Sketchers around LA. Your audience is smart, so if you say and promote things that don't align with your overall purpose and message, people will notice your inconsistencies and therefore trust you less and less.

Additionally, you must also balance your personality with the profession of nursing. We care for patients and work with other healthcare professionals. We are civil servants, and we have a duty to maintain the integrity of our profession. This is extremely important to remember as you engage online, select images to share (of both yourself and others), and interact in a manner that uplifts the profession and does not call its integrity into question.

This means that if you wouldn't write it, show it, or talk about it in front of your mom, preacher, patient, boss, or human resources managers, you probably shouldn't put it online. If a photo would make you blush, is it worth posting? Are you uplifting the profession or adding the hordes of negative stereotypes?

 Don't forget about HIPAA. You must remove any identifiable patient references from any of your stories. This even includes specific dates of care. Scramble your stories and ensure that the details are altered enough so they can never be tied back to a specific patient.

If you are a bedside nurse, and begin an online business that starts to flourish, it will gain attention not only from nurses, but from patients as well. If you share your opinion on very polarizing topics or post compromising photographs, you need to assume that patients or their loved ones may see it. You risk alienating them or making them feel uncomfortable. For example, if you post negative things about politicians, or other controversial topics like abortion, gun laws, and so forth, you risk (figuratively) cutting off the ears of people that may believe opposite of you. This does not mean you cannot have an opinion about the things you're passionate about (we just discussed how important it is to be you!), but the essential aspect of this is carefully deciding which topics to have a public opinion on, and then communicating it respectfully. You may find that even if people disagree with you, they will respect or even thank you for expressing your beliefs in a thoughtful and not in an aggressive or condescending manner. Therefore, if you want to discuss controversial topics, be selective. And also be ready for the opposing side of the topic to respond, potentially in less than gracious ways.

Therefore, when you post things on your blog or social media, remember that everyone can view it, even if they are not your intended audience. Not only are people watching what you say, they are also watching how you respond to people who disagree with you or who are rude to you. This includes current, former and future patients, colleagues, management, and administration.

Kati's personal experience

Once I was taking care of a patient and the CNA who was helping me clean the patient up casually mentioned one of my books. The patient's family member overheard him and asked about the book title and my writing. He immediately Googled me and pulled up my social media and asked, "Hey is that you!?" He was flipping through my website, Twitter and Instagram right in the patient's room. At that moment, I was very thankful for the mental screening process I go through each time I post something online. While it was a little odd to be in that position, I was comfortable with this patient's family member looking at my online presence. Had I posted something with derogatory language, overtly offensive, inappropriate, or compromising, I would have felt differently. The fact that patients can pull up my online platform instantly stays at the forefront of my mind. I do not want to give them any reason to question my integrity, or ability to care for them.

Remember, what you post online will not go away, even if you delete it. Someone may take a screenshot of your post before you remove it. If subpoenaed, social networks will supply that post. Once it's online, it might as well be written in stone.

You must be diligent in screening what you post. This can be a tough balance, because you also want to be authentic. If you are angry and frustrated about something and created a post, wait on it. Give yourself a day or so to feel and walk through your emotions. Then take a second look at it. You may have harnessed something important, and this anger and frustration is justified and has spurred you to inspire others or influence change. However, it is imperative to communicate this passion in a constructive way. This will ensure that you will maximize your reach and influence, and further solidify your authority, not make people question your ability to lead.

Get an Accountability Partner

Sometimes it's hard to notice when we've missed the mark, when we went too far, or when we're not following through with what we've said we would. Sometimes we put up a post that to us was edgy and funny, but we couldn't see how offensive it could have been. Or maybe we weigh in on a hot news topic, and didn't have all the facts. Or maybe a company has approached you about a contract, but their bottom line does not match up with yours. There are many instances in which it really helps to have the input of someone outside of the of the situation; but not someone so far outside of it that they don't know you, your values, your personality, your passion, and your purpose. Therefore, we highly encourage you to identify an accountability partner.

This accountability partner doesn't have to be a nurse. However, it should be someone who knows you personally, cares, and regularly reads your content. This may be a spouse, close friend, family member or colleague. Let them know your bottom line and your niche. Make sure it's someone whose judgment you trust; someone who will be honest with you and not just tell you what you want to hear.

If and when your platform develops, you may develop a fan-base. While this is a wonderful thing, it can also be a bit deceiving. You may post something that some people like, but is actually quite inappropriate or offensive and the only people responding are your fan-base cheering you on. All the while you may have actually completely changed what others (patients, professional organizations, businesses, colleagues, other members of the healthcare team, to name a few) think of you. A trusting and honest accountability partner is imperative because they will be honest with you in these instances. Sometimes we truly can't see how we're coming across and a constantly positive fan-base can blur our vision even more. Even some of the best communicators and leaders have mis-steps, post or say something that missed the mark, or said something in the wrong tone. People may hurt, think less of you, become offended, or isolated by your actions. They might even come right out and say it, publicly.

For every 50 people who tell you you're amazing, there may be a few thinking, "Oh wow, that is really not cool," and before you know it, you're missing out on professional opportunities and partnerships without even realizing it. Self-awareness is key, and an honest accountability partner can make a remarkable difference.

Empower your accountability partner to call you out when you're being inconsistent with your goals. Do not to respond negatively or defensively when they bring something up. Be approachable, be open, and be thankful for their investment and support. Run things by them before posting. Always have your bottom line as the priority. There may be opportunities that come which may provide some financial benefit, but if they don't align with your passion and purpose, it may end up not being worth it. Your account-ability partner may be able to see this before you do, and help you process these different opportunities in more of an objective manner.

CHAPTER 3

BRANDING
AND CONSISTENCY

A s we discussed earlier, your brand is the identity of your community and passion. Your community is rooted in your niche.

Think about a time you found a blog you enjoyed. Why did you enjoy it? What about it was particularly entertaining or helpful to you? Did you know the name of the person who built the site? Did you identify with them? Could you find related content on the blog?

Most people would say something along the lines of...

- The content was really relevant and helpful to me
- The content was easy to read and find
- I couldn't find this content anywhere else
- I thought this website was really easy to navigate and find more content
- I identify with the author
- I enjoy or appreciate the author's style
- I found what I needed quickly and didn't have to search any more
- I found more resources through related content

Did you try to find them on social media? If so, how did you go about finding them on social media?

Most people will take the blog name and just do a general search on that particular platform. For example, if I went to TheNerdy-Nurse.com and really enjoyed the content and decided I wanted to follow her on Twitter, I may click on her sidebar link to Twitter, or I may just go to my Twitter app and search "the nerdy nurse". If I cannot easily find her, I'll give up.

 Pro-tip: People have a short attention span. Everything needs an easy button.

After you have identified your niche and your passion, your brand will start to reveal itself to you. Having all these things decided and outlined will allow you to present a much more cohesive image to your audience.

Establishing your brand is essential. Even if you're in the beginning stages of blogging, you need to make clear who you are and what you're about. You, as the community leader, will appear to have everything together, and your brand is easily identified.

Determining the Type of Brand

The first question you must ask yourself is if your brand centered around you and your name, or if it will be more of a business brand with you behind it.

For example, Nurse Alice is a brand based upon her as a person. Her logo has her name it in, her blog is her writing posts about health and wellness, as well as different ways she is engaged in the media, and educating people on those topics. Nurse Alice's brand is Nurse Alice.

Elizabeth Scala is another nurse whose brand is built upon her as a person. Her website is elizabethscala.com, and while "Nursing From Within" is her tagline and writing about burnout is her focus, it still is her providing education and information. Elizabeth Scala's brand is Elizabeth Scala.

Jon Haws at NRSNG is a nurse who has built a business brand. While he is the nurse behind NRSNG and a face you frequently see throughout posts and the website, he is not NRSNG. NRSNG is the brand, not Jon Haws.

Let's be clear in saying that there is not a correct or incorrect answer here. The best choice is definitely dependent upon your ultimate goals.

Your branding, including your URL and related social media names, will make an impact on how people perceive your content and your ability to scale your online presence and related business.

If you are the brand...

Pros	Cons
• Phenomenal name recognition • People become interested in learning about you as a person • Potential for more speaking events • Professional credibility to your audience and leaders in the industry • You only have to maintain one set of social media profiles • Can be easier to establish credibility and expertise as a person • Can lead to faster professional advancement	• Less options for logos, design • If you want to step away or stop, it's not something you can transfer to another person • Less options for lateral moves, not related to nursing • Potentially gender polarizing - for example, men may not want to wear a "Nurse Sarah" t-shirt • May be hard to differentiate between business you and personal you • Difficulty scaling content and your mission • Likely cannot sell site/brand

If your business is the brand...

Pros	Cons
• Potential for more business opportunities… businesses love working with other businesses • Ability to differentiate your personal self from your business online • Easier to sell it one day and since your name is not an integral aspect of this, you'll be able have a smoother transition out for potentially more money • Easier to scale your business by taking on writers and other staff • Can be seen as more legitimate in the business world	• Nurses will trust other nurses over a business or corporate entity. You'll lose some of that trust factor. • If you also desire to do speaking engagements, you may need to create an additional website or space for interested parties • May need to manage separate social media accounts for the business

Name and Tagline

Next, you should decide what you want your brand to be called. As you do this, you must research your options. Complete a comprehensive search to see if people have your desired website name, various social handles, any trademarks, and close misspellings.

If you do want your name as your brand, you must know there are many who have chosen to do this, so your selection may be limited. Nurse Mendoza, Nurse Alice, Nurse Beth, Nurse Nacole, Nurse Jackie, Nurse Mo, Nurse Gail, and even Nurse Golytely are all spoken for already.

If you want to build a brand, check out different nursing brands out there and get a lay of the land.

You want to have a sharable name because you will become known more quickly if people are sharing your content. People must not be embarrassed to share your brand on their social platforms. If you have a curse word in your brand, if it's negative, or inappropriate, you may immediately cause many to disengage.

Also, while most of the profession is female, there is a quickly growing aspect that is male. Keep this in mind. If you have a website, handle, or design that has overwhelmingly traditional feminine style (flowers, pinks, hearts, bows), you may turn off that aspect of your audience, or prevent them from sharing your content.

Deciding on a tagline is also important. A tagline is another word for a slogan or catchphrase. I know it sounds a little car-salesman like to create a slogan, but it's essential for someone to hear or see your brand name, and within just a few words, know what it's about.

Here are a few examples:

- FreshRN - Growing New Nurses
- NRSNG - Creating Nurses
- Elizabeth Scala - Nursing from Within
- Nurse.com - Oncourse Learning
- Donna Cardillo - The Inspiration Nurse
- Nurse Mendoza - The YouTube Nurse
- The Nerdy Nurse - Nursing's Leading Technology Voice
- NNBA - #1 Nurse Business Owner Network

Appearance

In this ever-evolving field, it's important to have a visually appealing brand. You want people to enjoy looking at, engaging with, and sharing your content. One of the reasons people love to share things is because it looks, or actually is, cool. You could have good content, but if it's living on a website that has an odd color combination, is poorly organized, and takes time to figure out how to navigate, people are less likely to engage and share. We want to pull people in, provide value, and engage them so much so that not only do they want to come back for more, but also they want to share it with their friends.

Trends evolve quickly so it's important to be tuned into what the top and fast-growing brands are doing. We highly recommend following brands you find that you really enjoy, nursing and non-nursing alike, and try to figure out what you like about them, and put your own spin on it. Have other people look at your logo, tagline, social media platforms, and ask about their first impressions.

Please do not hold onto your brand with white knuckles. Knowing when to pivot is an essential aspect of staying relevant.

Remember back in 2002 when everyone was obsessed with the Comic Sans font? Soon, it became the bane of the existence of many and people started to loathe that font. Those whose websites and blogs were slathered in Comic Sans quickly lost credibility with many, as the popularity of that font quickly plummeted and people equated it with immaturity. Remember, people share things because they think are *cool*. What someone shares on a social media page is a reflection of themselves So if you show your logo to people and their first thought is that it's a bit young or childish, you may want to rethink your approach.

Think about what's easy to read. We've been to blogs before that had a yellow background, blue words, and purple links. We've also been to websites where we can't figure out who is actually writing the content, how to navigate to older posts, or we couldn't find their content because there were so many ads on the page, we couldn't tell which was which.

Try to think like your target audience at all times, making their consumption of your content as smooth and easy as possible. You want them to enjoy visiting your site, checking out your content, and signing up for your mailing list. You want them to come back. Bonus points if you can wow them enough to share your information with their peer group, which would also fit into your target audience.

Your Logo and Branding Kit

An important part of the appearance of your blog and brand is the logo. Your logo captures your style, your color scheme, and the overall tone of your brand. For example, if you have a cartoon version of yourself included in your logo, your audience will assume your brand is fun and casual. They'll also associate it with you as an individual. On the flip side, if your brand is stylized text, clean and modern, and calming colors, your audience will be inclined to associate it as a hip and modern professional company. Either of these is acceptable, of course. It just depends on what you are looking for.

Creating a logo is one of the first things that you should consider hiring someone to complete. The good news is that it typically not expensive. You can get a logo designed by someone on Fiverr or

UpWork for less than $100. Around $25-50 is fair for a simple logo based on text and vectors and not requiring any drawing.

When you get your logo complete it's a good idea to get a couple different sizes done. First, you'll get your main logo done with a size that fits your theme header (more on themes later). Then you'll need a square version 250x250 for social media icons. You can also get Facebook and Twitter headers complete. Often getting these all done up by the same person will create a more consistent look and be much more cost effective.

 Pro-tip: Ask for a version of your logo with a transparent background so you can use it to watermark photos. You can also pay a few bucks extra to get the source file so small tweaks can be made later, if needed.

When you develop your logo, you'll select the colors and style of fonts to utilize. This will become your color scheme and you should make a note of all the hex codes for the colors used and the font in a single location (a Word or Google Doc is recommended). This document, along with your logo will be your branding kit. You can sometimes use the same font on your blog to really tie the branding together. Of course, this depends on how easy the font is to read and the look overall. Readability is far more important than font consistency.

Having a branding kit will be a big benefit as you build out your site. You'll have clear guidelines for the color scheme and options for font choices for any designers that you hire. They'll be thankful for the clear direction and you'll be thankful for the great results.

Your logo and color scheme will not last forever. Sooner or later your market will change, your message will evolve, and you'll fall out of love with your original choice for logo and colors. The great news is that by the time you get there you'll likely be earning revenue and be able to spend more money to get something amazing. The cycle will then repeat. Changing the branding every three to five years is not uncommon. We've both changed our branding and logo. It means you're growing, and that's great!

Kati's Brand Story

I started out with an anonymous Tumblr blog, and decided to name it "Nurse Eye Roll". I couldn't get that nurse name out of my mind and just went with it. I didn't start the blog with any intentions of making it a business. I just wanted a place to share my funny nurse stuff and little posts I wrote. I wanted it to be anonymous because I was scared of getting fired and didn't really understand what I could and could not say on social media.

It quickly grew and people were sharing my content regularly. I then created a website, a Twitter handle, and a Pinterest page with the same name.

Things continued to grow as I started to create articles and submit them to various nursing sites. I think nurses really identified with the "Nurse Eye Roll" name because so many of us at the bedside have that eye-rolling experience. Early on, I connected with Brittney after really enjoying her blog. She advised me to really think about that brand and if it's something I wanted plastered everywhere, as some people may view that name as sarcastic or that I'm making fun of patients. While I understood what she meant, I felt like I still wanted to continue with that brand at that time. I also realized that I had sort of hit the glass ceiling of being anonymous and Brittney encouraged me to come out of proverbial anonymous nursing blog closet.

I decided to stay as "Nurse Eye Roll", but to no longer be anonymous. I cleaned up some of the more edgy posts I had made as an anonymous brand, then talked to my manager about my intentions. After getting her emphatic support, I put my name to my brand.

I had a profile picture of a nurse rolling her eyes and my "Nurse Eye Roll" name, but then started to have my real name and face on my website. I did a professional photo shoot and uploaded those pictures on my site. I eventually created my first logo with the help of a graphic designer, decided on a color palette, and updated the website in early 2015. While I was happy with how it looked, I just didn't have a total peace with my brand name.

Looking back, I should have heeded Brittney's advice. While many nurses loved, and identified with the "Nurse Eye Roll" name, it was quite a turnoff for some individuals, and a major turn off for businesses. Not many people wanted to publicize that they were working with someone named "Nurse Eye Roll". I spoke with someone at a company I'd worked with for a few years, and they expressed that they did experience some hesitancy to work with me based off of the name. Once they saw my work, they really valued it, but had someone not really explained what I was about, I could have missed out on some major opportunities.

I decided that not only did I want to rebrand, but I also wanted to narrow my niche. I decided to focus on the specific area of nursing that was truly my passion: new nurses. I came up with a new brand, FreshRN, and sat down with a few graphic artists and got my new logo, tagline, and website built. I decided to create a website/resource hub solely for the new graduate nurse, and a separate site (katikleber.com) for parties interested in speaking events, or working with me directly rather than the brand.

I let my audience know of my transition, and then started turning my social platforms into ones that coincided with what I was now doing. Since the change, I've had more interest in ad sales, sponsored posts, and inquiries from some of the largest professional nursing organizations in the country.

While Nurse Eye Roll served its purpose at the time and I will miss that brand, I know FreshRN is not only a better move, but serves my passion more directly.

Brittney's Brand Story

I jumped into the world of social media as a coping mechanism due to the bullying I experienced as a new nurse. I started on Twitter anonymously tweeting frustrations and occasional highlights of my experiences as a new nurse. I'd spend my lunch breaks with my nurse friends on Twitter learning and growing through a newfound community.

I went through a few different names including NurseBrittney, AmusingNurse, and NurseMusings. I also started a blog around the same time (2009) for my nursing commentary that required more than 140 characters.

I blogged about nursing, technology, my life, and whatever came to mind. I realized that "Nurse Brittney" wasn't super catchy, and actually probably was too transparent making it easy for me to be identified. I wasn't quite ready for that.

When thinking through the type of content I wanted to appear on my blog, I thought of the name "The Nerdy Nurse." I enjoyed the alliteration, the term nerd, and the breadth of topics that could be covered by a name like that. I bought the URL TheNerdyNurse.com, updated my then BlogSpot blog to point to that URL. I focused my content to more nursing and technology and really worked to provide value in the nursing community. I changed my Twitter handle to @TheNerdyNurse and continued to blog anonymously for another year.

I would have likely continued to blog anonymously had I not been approached by a small tech blog to work as a contributing editor. This opportunity came with several perks that were appealing, but the requirement was that I use my real photo and my real name. This hit me like a ton of bricks at the time. I had never considered doing this.

Thinking of coming out of the blogging closet was scary. I was afraid of what might happen if one of my colleagues, or worse my boss, happened to stumble across it. Would I be written up? Would I be fired? Could I lose my license? Was what I was doing against some policy somewhere? Should I even be blogging at all?

After quite a bit of soul searching, I decided that even though my blogging had started as a mechanism to cope with my poor experience, it had evolved into a valuable source of nursing information that I could (with a little effort) take pride in.

I performed an in-depth blog and social media audit and removed any and all questionable materials. Any stories that could be even remotely identifiable were scrambled and details changed. Even though I was confident that most of the nurses I worked with didn't even know what the internet was, I wanted to be sure my livelihood and their feelings were protected.

Once I was confident that The Nerdy Nurse was a brand I could stand behind, I added my name and photo to my blog and I took the editor position at the tech blog. This has been one the best decisions I have made in my nursing and blogging journey. It empowered me to include The Nerdy Nurse on my resume. Having a blog made me feel more confident as a nurse. It was also was one of the primary reasons I was able to glide into informatics without a master's degree. This experience cemented the value of blogging to my nursing career.

I sometimes struggle with the fact that The Nerdy Nurse isn't just the name of a site, it's also seamlessly identifiable with me as an individual. I'm not just the owner of the site; I'm the physical embodiment of the brand. This creates considerably more pressure on my own personal brand. It also means that it would be nearly impossible to sell the brand as it would be difficult to disassociate me from it. When people think of The Nerdy Nurse they think of Brittney Wilson.

Content and focus on the blog has evolved, but generally the brand has had the same mission. The focus is on nursing and technology. The Nerdy Nurse provides resources to help nurses feel more empowered, informed, and live a better life. It became clear that stories about my family, travel, or general lifestyle topics that did not have anything to do with nursing or technology were less valuable, so I no longer write about those topics.

A good brand is always evolving to meet the needs of their customers. The Nerdy Nurse seeks to do the same. It has changed and will change as the audience evolves. It will follow the needs of nurses and nursing students with a focus of providing solutions, but it will also align with my passions and goals.

CHAPTER 4

HOW TO
START A BLOG

"There are 100 million blogs in the world, and it's part of my job as the co-founder of WordPress to help many more people start blogging."

- Matt Mullenweg

Buckle up baby. We're gonna get nerdy! Once you've decided you want to blog, the next step is to actually build one. Over the years, we've made our share of mistakes and want to save you the trial and tribulation of searching the web to find every detail. While we won't go into a large amount of technical detail, this chapter will give you an overview of exactly what you need to do to have your blog up in running in a short period of time.

Pick Your Platform (Hint: WordPress)

When you decide you want to blog, it's important to consider the end goal. Are you just looking for a place to share your knowledge or thoughts with the world? Are you looking to attract clients to a new or existing business? Are you looking to blog as a form of income? The answer to each question can impact your choice for platform or content management system (CMS).

For example, if you already have a website where you provide goods or services, you should add your blog to this website on the same domain. Specifically, you should ensure this blog isn't on a sub-domain (blog.yourdomain.com) but instead is on the same domain. It can perhaps be segmented by a category (yourdomain. com/blog/). If you create your blog as a subdomain Google will actually see your blog as a separate site for your main website thus losing a lot of the value of having a blog in the first place.

For most purposes, WordPress will fit the bill. It's the most popular CMS on the web powering more than 27% of websites[2]. It is an open-source (free) software that allows you to publish content easily. The primary benefit of the WordPress is it's fairly easy to use, has tons of standard plugins and add-ons, and generally performs well in search.

For simplicity (and because in our opinion, it's the best), the rest of this chapter will be referring to WordPress. However, much of the information can be applied to the content management system of your choice.

WordPress.com Versus WordPress.Org (Self-hosted)

It's important to understand that there is a difference between building a site by going to WordPress.com and starting a free account versus buying your own domain and uploading/activating a copy of self-hosted WordPress (WordPress.org). WordPress.com limits your ability to monetize your content and has less flexibility than hosting your own content and simply using the WordPress platform on your own domain. The term self-hosted simply means that you own the hosting and domain that the WordPress platform is served from.

The decision between WordPress.com and WordPress.org is really a no brainer. With Wordpress.com you are locked into using approved themes and plugins. You can buy a domain name, but there are other considerations. For example, you may go over the allotted free data limit, which will come with an additional fee. You'll also have to manage your domain email on a separate provider. More importantly, WordPress.com can shut you down at any time and

---

2 K. Karol. "The Ultimate List Of WordPress Statistics". *CodeinWP Blog*. N.p., 2017. Web. 23 Mar. 2017.

remove all your content if they perceive you have violated their terms of service (TOS) [3,4].

The basic difference is just where the site/content is hosted, but it can make some forms of monetization complicated. If you think you'll ever use your blog to earn any form of income, save yourself some trouble and start your blog using your own domain and hosting and use the self-hosted version of WordPress.

Hosting

In order for your blog to be accessible to the world it will need to be served up to the world by a host. A website or blog host is the company that provides the technical architecture to house your content online. In short, they have a server that they'll allow you to place your content on and ensure that it gets served up when people land on your little corner of the web. Different website hosts support and optimize for different types of CMS.

WordPress is typically served on these types of hosting plans:

- Shared Hosting
- Managed Hosting
- Dedicated Hosting

Shared hosting means that your blog content and database is hosted on a server with hundreds of other blogs. For most new bloggers, shared hosting is a good choice because it's affordable and your traffic will be low. However, if one of the sites on a shared host is particularly demanding, your performance may suffer. If you discover that you have performance or plugin issues that won't resolve, shared hosting may be the culprit.

Examples:

- Host Gator
- Bluehost
- Go Daddy

Managed hosting is typically the same basic format as shared hosting. However, these hosts optimize their servers specifically for WordPress and do a much better job of managing overall server load. This yields a better performance at a cost that is usually only

---

3 Brinker, Mark. "7 Little-Known Reasons Wordpress.Com Sucks For Serious Bloggers • Smart Blogger". *Smart Blogger*, 2017, https://smartblogger.com/wordpress-hosting/.
4 "Terms Of Service". *Wordpress.Com*, 2017, http://en.wordpress.com/tos.

slightly higher. Often, managed hosts will provide basic site updates and maintenance for you as well. If you have more than 50,000 visitors each month, or are experiencing performance issues on a shared host, managed hosting is a good option.

Examples:
- Lightning Base
- Site Ground
- WP Engine
- DreamHost
- Pagely

Dedicated hosting involves a hosting your blog on a private server. This can be a virtual server or a physical server completely devoted to your site. Your level of support will vary based upon the host. Many offer concierge type services to make the management of your blog much easier. Some, however, offer little support and are not optimized for WordPress. If you experience performance issues on a managed host or have a large amount of traffic (over 200,000 visitors) a dedicated host may be worth exploring.

Examples:
- Wired Tree
- VPS Net

You will install the WordPress CMS on the host of your choice typically using integrated tools provided by your host. This will be done in an administrator area called cPanel. Check your host for their specific instructions on how to do so.

cPanel: A control panel that includes automation tools, software installation, and settings for websites.

Attaching Your Domain Name to Your Host

When setting up your blog you may already own a domain. If this is the case, you will need to go to the registrar for your domain and adjust the nameservers to point to your host. Don't worry if you If you haven't purchased a domain before selecting a host. Often, a domain name will be included for free and you will not have to go through the extra step.

Domain name registrars:

- Name Cheap
- Go Daddy

Make it Pretty with an Awesome Theme

Once you load WordPress on your host, you'll want to make it pretty with a theme. In fact, the ability to easily load a new theme, that can change the entire appearance of your website, is one of the best features of WordPress. With a new theme, you can quickly customize your blog and make it beautiful with an off-the-shelf theme.

Theme: A group of code that changes the appearance and style of your site. This can include fonts, colors, formatting, and layouts.

The available styles of a theme are as broad as you can possibly imagine. No matter what type of content you are producing, you can find something that matches your brand and vision.

Paid, Free, and Custom Themes

There are thousands of free themes available for WordPress that will meet the needs of most bloggers starting out. There's no right or wrong type of theme to use as long as it has a decent amount of positive reviews and fulfills your design needs.

Premium, or paid, themes usually offer upgraded theme features such increased customization choices, a structure that is built for SEO, and custom add-ons called plugins (more on that later) developed specifically to work with that theme provided. These often enhance the experience and provide a cleaner, more polished, look. Prices for paid themes range for as little as $20 to as high as $400 for an off-the-shelf theme.

Great premium themes include:

- All StudioPress themes, including Genesis
- Divi by Elegant Themes

If you have trouble finding a free or premium theme to meet your unique needs, you can always opt to have a theme developed or customized for you. To do this you'll typically partner with a WordPress designer who will assess your needs and align with your vision to create and install a custom theme specific to you. The price for this service ranges from $500 to over $10,000. One risk in working with a designer and developing a custom theme is the need to maintain that relationship in the event updates in the WordPress platform make your custom theme incompatible. This should not deter you from this path, but is something to consider.

Customizing Your Own Theme

If you happen to find a theme that you like, but need to alter it slightly, you can do so fairly easily using Cascading Style Sheets (CSS). This is a simple coding language that can allow you to make tweaks to appearance for items such as fonts, color, and general formatting. This is an intermediate skill that should be explored after you've established a general understanding of WordPress and blogging. There are many written tutorials available on the web as well as videos on YouTube. Some themes, such as those in StudioPress, even have dedicated training related to customizing your theme via CSS.

CSS: Cascading Style Sheets is a markup language that deals with the style and representation of your website. CSS impacts your fonts, colors, size and locations of tables and DIVs.

Widgets

Customizing WordPress is fairly easy. While the general look and style of your blog is managed through the theme, adding specific functions and features to the sidebar, below content, and other locations are typically handled by widgets. These widgets allow you to easily pop content into specific locations using html, short-codes, or plugins. The widgets section in WordPress allows you to drag and drop different elements like post categories, recent content and comments, social sharing icons, or contact forms.

Plugins

After you've installed a theme you'll want to utilize add-ons specific to WordPress that allow you to quickly and easily insert things into your blog without needing to use HTML or other coding. These add-ons for WordPress are called plugins. There are thousands of plugins available to complete a variety of functions. Many of them are free, but paid (or premium) plugins are available for more complex functionality.

Examples of the types of things that plugins can do include:

- Easily adding beautiful sharing icons to your posts
- Displaying a feed of your most recent Pinterest pins or tweets on your sidebar
- Integrating your mailing list provider to easily add opt-in forms to your posts
- Tracking traffic through external tools like Google Analytics
- Optimizing your content for search

Plugins are an essential aspect of your website and have the potential to make the site look sharp, streamlined, and easier for both you and your audience to enjoy.

Recommended Plugins

Comment Management

Recommended: Akismet Anti-Spam

Price: FREE

This popular comment moderation tool helps to prevent your blog from being overwhelmed by spam or fake comments.

Social Sharing

Recommended: Easy Social Sharing

Price: $27 one-time

This highly customizable social sharing plugin allows you to place social share icons in just about any location you can imagine. It includes fan counters to display your followers on various social media platforms that can easily be displayed in in a widget on your sidebar. You can also view which post has the most social shares via an integrated dashboard.

Search Engine Optimization

Recommended: Yoast SEO

Price: FREE (Premium available)

This popular plugin helps guide you to create content that will easily rank in search engines to get more organic traffic from Google. It works by ensuring that your focus keyword is included in the correct locations in content as well as well as checking for SEO functions on images, titles, and the slug (URL) of the post. You can also enable Google Analytics and Webmaster tools using this plugin. However, Google Tag Manager (discussed below), is recommended for integrating Google products.

List Building

Recommended: Thrive Leads

Price: $47 (Or recurring if bundled)

This plugin allows the ability to build beautiful, custom opt-in forms that can be placed in a variety of places on your blog. This can be a bar at the top of the page or a box with a free-offer at the end of your post. A great feature is that you can customize which opt-in forms appear based on the post category or tags.

Integration of Google Tools

Recommended: Google Tag Manager

Price: FREE

Google Tag Manager allows you to easily store the code for Google Analytics, Google Search Console, Google AdSense, and other non-Google scripts in an external location that can be called upon by your host to generate related code upon a page load. This can reduce the need to manually add codes to areas within WordPress. It is also usually better for the overall health of your site as it lessens the strain of having an individual plugin for each of these functions or separate lines of code for each of these actions.

While your blog can function without these plugins, we highly recommend investing a little time and (in some case) money into them. If you're serious about blogging, they will be well worth the investment.

Analytics and Data Tracking

In you want to create a successful blog, focusing on analytics is a must. While blogging at its core is built upon creating powerful, emotional content that provides value to readers, there are key practices that must be observed for long term success. Analytics will help ensure that people are finding your content and completing specific actions. For example, if you write a post about your favorite books for nurses, a natural desire is for people who find that post to purchase one or all of your recommendations.

Analytics tools, especially Google Analytics and Google Search Console, provide insight into how a person found your content, what they did once they got there, and what they did when they were finished. In short, these tools help you track the complete path that a user takes when consuming your content. It will also show your most popular content, search terms, and referral sources. With additional manipulation, Google Analytics can also show you where a reader went after leaving your blog. This can be useful to track conversions for products or services you've recommended.

To clarify, Google Analytics can show you which posts or pages have the most the most traffic and where they came from. When integrated with Google Webmaster tools it can also provide a sampling of the keywords that users searched for to find your specific content.

Post and Pages

There are two main types of content contained within a WordPress site: posts and pages. Each serve a distinct purpose and should be utilized accordingly. When trying to determine whether a post or page should be used, you should think about how often, if ever, it will be updated and referenced. Posts, for example, are typically published and not typically changed on a routine basis. Pages, however, are frequently referenced and constantly evolve as your site evolves.

Posts

Blog posts, or posts, are what will account for the majority of the content of your blog. A good blog post has a minimum of 300 words, includes subheadings, a captivating title, and solves a specific problem or explores a specific topic. There are dozens of different types of posts that you could write. The website DigitalMarketer.com has a resource called The Ultimate List of Blog Post Ideas[5] that groups posts into a few basic categories.

Post types are grouped according to purpose and then a type within that purpose. The purposes include:

- Be Useful
- Be Generous
- Be Entertaining
- Be Timely
- Be Human
- Be Promotional
- Be Controversial
- Be Engaging

For example, if you want to write a post that is useful, you might consider writing a how-to, case study, list, or even an ultimate guide post. If you want to be human, you might write something inspirational, a professional rant, or something where you really let your guard down and get very intimate with your audience.

How Often Should You Publish?

One of the biggest questions in blogging is "How often should I publish?"

There's really no wrong or right answer to this. Whether you publish once a week, twice a week, every day, or twice a month, there's really no wrong or right answer to this. What's more important is that you pick a schedule and stick with it. Your readers will appreciate your consistency and Google loves websites with content that is updated routinely.

---

5 The Ultimate List Of Blog Post Ideas". *DigitalMarketer*. N.p., 2015. Web. 23 Mar. 2017.

Pages

Pages are created to store static content that is generally informational about a site and its purpose. Pages can also be used as table of contents type resources outlining the best or most desirable content related to a similar topic.

 Pro-tip: Create a page that is a list of resources related to products or services that you recommend. Link to related posts with further detail. Include affiliate links where available. This will be a post that you can reference and link to often so it will be a valuable, high-traffic page, that can be a money maker as well.

Every blog should have a few key pages to provide the best possible user experience. These are outlined below.

About

An About Page is a location to summarize the overall purpose of your blog as well as the author or team of authors creating the content. The style and specific content will vary based upon whether you are writing as a personal brand or company brand. Generally, it will include mission-type statements describing the purpose of the site and what someone can learn by using it. If a personal brand is associated, even if not the primary focus, there is usually a short biography as well.

Disclaimers

Your disclaimers page should inform your audience that any actions based upon information provided on your site is done so at their own risk. The general setup and flow of this page can be up to you, but it is recommended[6] that you address the following subjects:

- Terms of use
- Copyright policy
- HIPAA policy
- Readers will hold author harmless

---

6 Krook, Nienke. "How To Write A Disclaimer For Your Blog | The Travel Tester". *The Travel Tester.* N.p., 2012. Web. 23 Mar. 2017.

- Privacy statement
- Advertisers, sponsors, and affiliates relationships and terms

Provide information here that will protect you and your brand legally regarding any information provided on your blog. Be sure to clearly define that nothing should be considered legal or medical advice and that professional recommendations are your opinions only.

Contact

A contact page should be included to allow your audience to easily connect with you. This page should include a contact form rather than an email address. This will help control spam. You can also set up specific options for different types of communication forms. For example, you can have a subject related to sponsorship or requests to guest post on your site. The free plugin Contact Form 7[7] is simple, yet highly customizable and allows radio buttons, drop-downs, and text fields to create forms for just about anything you need. The responses are automatically sent to your email and you can reply directly via email.

Products and Services

Be sure to include a page that lists all the products and services you offer. This may be info products such as books or courses, professional services such as coaching, or any physical products you create. Listing these items on one page provides your audience with a quick resource to know all the services you have to offer. This makes things easier for your audience. It also increases the potential that your readers will buy from you if they see all you have to offer in a central location.

Awards and Mentions (Press)

As you grow in your brand or business, you will no doubt receive press, awards, and mentions on other websites. It's a great idea to keep a running list of these mentions to further provide legitimacy to your value. Chose a simple structure to organize and keep this page updated often. If you are asked to provide proof of your notoriety, this is an excellent resource.

---

7 "Contact Form 7". *WordPress.org*. N.p., 2017. Web. 23 Mar. 2017.

Testimonials

If you provide a specific product or service, such as speaking or teaching, a testimonial page is recommended. Use this page to display quotes citing the quality of your work. If you do not have any testimonials to include, request those as soon as possible. Wait to create this page until you have enough to mention.

Pro-tip: When you provide any of your services ask your client to write a recommendation for you on LinkedIn. This provides a validated record of your service and you can easily copy the comments to include on your testimonial page on your blog.

Other Pages That May Be Helpful

- Advertising and Sponsorship - This page should outline your general terms regarding advertising and sponsorship. You can also choose to link to your media kit and rates here or include a contact form to request additional information.

- Writing Portfolio - If part of your business includes freelance writing, it is helpful to have a single page listing your work on other sites. Every time you get content published on a site besides your own (paid or otherwise) include a link and brief description on this page.

- Disclosure - You should disclose any financial relationship you have. If a specific post is sponsored, the disclosure for that should be within that post. However, if your site has a sponsor or if you have a partnership you address across multiple channels, you should list that relationship on a disclosure page.

- Blog - If your WordPress site is built as a portfolio; you'll want to have a blog page that acts as a running list of your blog content.

Menus

In order for your blog to be functional to your readers, you'll need to ensure that your menus are user-friendly and intuitive. Your menus should include pages you have created and potentially links to blog categories as well. Depending on the theme you have, you may have one or two menu locations. Also, each menu item can have a sub menu, allowing you to organize your content in a way that makes things easy to find. You can usually use space on your menu to a search box or social icons. Typically, you can only include one or the other, so choose based upon which is more valuable to your audience.

If you have a single menu, use one menu option for your blog. You can also include sub-menus for your categories. If you have a second menu, it's beneficial to use it for content categories. You'll only have room for 5-8, so if you have more you'll want to choose your most popular/profitable. You can also include an archive page that shows your most recent posts, most popular posts, and a list of all categories.

Suggested Menu Layout

Home	About	Contact	Services	Products	Blog	Search

Categories and Tags

When writing content, you want to ensure that it can easily be found by readers. Many people will come to your site and read one article, not exploring or ever returning. There are several factors that contribute to this, but the primary cause is that they are not engaged. This may mean that your content isn't great, your site is slow to load, or they cannot find what they are looking for. Having a clear and well-utilized tagging and categorization system on your blog can make the difference between a website visitor that stays on your site or bounces after one page.

Categories

If you think of your blog like a book, categories are the chapters. Typically, you want to keep the number of categories fairly small and focused on your specific niche. For example, if you have a nursing blog focusing on the ED your categories could include Patient Care Tips, Career Advice, Clinical Resources, and Funny ED Stories. There's no set number of categories you can have, but you should keep it under 20. A good number seems to be 8-12. Consider that if all categories are listed on a page (like your archive page), you want them to be unique enough and clear enough that if someone clicks on that category they know exactly what type of content they are going to get.

If possible, planning categories from the beginning is helpful in planning content and ensuring you're staying on brand/niche. However, you can grow as you go along without issue. One mistake to avoid is using categories as tags. Generally, blog posts should only fit in one or two categories, while they may have many tags. If you find that you're using more than three categories on every post, you may want to consider converting those categories to tags.

Good content management including proper use of tagging and categories is helpful for multiple reasons. While it does have some impact on SEO, it's generally minor. It's much more beneficial in the overall organization of content. Tagging is also utilized in plugins that recommended similar content. If someone really likes an article you wrote about a particular topic and want to know more, they can click on the related tag or related content referred to them by a recommended content plugin.

Tags

So now that you're thinking of your blog like a book, let's take it one step further. Imagine your blog is a textbook. All good textbooks have an index to help you locate specific terms and topics. Unlike book chapters (or blog categories), which are few and broad, there can be thousands of words and phrases listed in a book's index. With a blog, it's exactly the same with tags. There can be hundreds or even thousands of tags.

Categories and Tagging Example

A good example of this is in some content on The Nerdy Nurse around HIPAA and data privacy. While the topic of HIPAA is on niche, it's also very specific and not a primary topic Brittney writes about frequently. She does write about technology often, and it fits perfectly within the Gadgets & Technology category. There is enough content and it is something specific enough that she would also tag it with HIPAA or even HIPAA violations.

CHAPTER 5

CREATE AMAZING
CONTENT

*"(Brand storytelling) isn't about pushing advertising,
it's about bringing value"*

- Gary Vee

N ow that you have a blog with a good logo, tagline, feel
good about how it looks, and how things work behind the
scenes, let's talk about what people are really coming to
see: your content.

Your content doesn't just have to be blog posts; it can also be
video and podcasts. However, a classic blog based on your writing
and images is the fastest way to get started. As you grow with your
blog and your brand you can, and should, consider expanding
your reach by creating different types of media to complement
your blog.

Important Things to Consider as You Blog

Remember how we said earlier that people are easily distracted?
People want what they came for quickly and efficiently, or they'll
be gone never to return before you know it. Emerson Spartz the

of CEO of Dose.com said, "Write like you're getting paid a million dollars for every word you delete."

The more concise, the better.

Now, please don't misunderstand us here. We don't want you to have a 50-word post. The take home point is to not spend 500 words describing something that could have been expressed in 75. Whenever content starts to ramble, over-explains, or is just plain boring, people stop reading, tune out, and move on. Make sure every word and sentence is valuable and necessary.

Additionally, people don't like to read huge paragraphs at a time. People consume more content with shorter sentences and smaller blocks of words. Also, if your reader loses their place, it's easier to find it again within a few lines rather than within a large chunk of text.

When in doubt, go to the next line.

People also want transitions in content to be easily identifiable. This is where headings come into play. Use as many as are needed to outline the transitions in the content. Your readers (and Google) will love you for this.

When you write a blog, don't get bogged down in your past experiences with writing from school. You aren't turning it in for a grade. No one is going to check your APA. In fact, if you cite things in APA it's going to feel sterile and boring. Your inexperience with blogging will be painfully obvious. Cite sources throughout your content by linking the actual words of the post. No one wants to scroll to the bottom to get to the sources.

As nurses, we're familiar with the term "best practices". A similar term can be applied to blogging and that's, "most effective practices". You want to be as effective and efficient as possible in your posts. Let's talk about some common blogging mistakes people make, and with each mistake, we'll identify an effective practice to replace it with.

Blogging Mistake #1 - Your Posts are Too Long

Remember the importance of being concise? We have seen blog posts that were upwards of 1K words that could have communicated the same message just as effectively in 400 words.

As writers, sometimes we get inspired, think we have an eloquent way to word it or a unique perspective, and get passionate and pumped. Our fingers fiercely pound our chicklet keyboards with the furry of 10,000 nurses who are late on their charting. We write epic blog posts and feel extremely proud of ourselves. If we're good bloggers, we wait a day and review the content. Then when considering the overall purpose of the post and we determine it doesn't necessarily align with our brand or bottom line. Being married to an idea that sounded good at first and trying to force it to work when it simply doesn't work wastes time of creates useless content. When reading through it on a second pass, you'll likely find that you can safely eliminate half of a passionately written post.

Most effective practice: Have a word count goal

There isn't a magic word count number, as these recommendations tend to change. However, a total of 500 words is a good place to start. Some people write 1000-2000 word posts. As long as there are images, headings, and really valuable content, people will stay engaged. Most blog posts do not require so many words to get the message across. One thousand words is quite a long time to keep a reader's attention. Most likely, people aren't reading all of it.

Finally, you can get away with a large master post (7-8K words), if you're filling it with tons of links, images, headings, resources, videos, and audio content. You could break these into several posts with a single master post connecting all the related content together. Either method takes quite a bit of time and planning to create effectively and must serve a specific purpose with appropriate SEO (more on that later).

Blogging Mistake #2 - Your Posts Don't Have Headings

Headings help to break up text and compartmentalize content into bite-sized nuggets which makes it easier to consume. Headings and sub-headings act as an outline for your content. Typically, a blog post is structured by having a few intro sentences, 2-4 headings with a few paragraphs underneath, images throughout, and followed by a few conclusion sentences. These headings allow people who are skimming to see what you'll be talking about and when. It also lets Google know the main focuses of the content. So, make sure your headings actually describe the subject matter of the paragraphs that it is heading.

Pro-tip: Use headings to break up content with real descriptions of the content that follows it. Do not use headings for style. Create custom CSS for that.

Let's take a look at one of Brittney's most popular posts: How to Pass the NCLEX with 75 Questions in One Attempt. This is just a screenshot of one aspect of the post, which is much longer than what you see here. She's got her content broken up in multiple paragraphs with great headings.

Don't Study On Your NCLEX Test Day

Just don't study on test day. You aren't going to find some magical formula on how to pass the NCLEX the day of your test. You'll just end up stressing yourself out if you try to cram in "just a few more questions." We've already discussed how at this point you really shouldn't be attempting to cram in content. Try to find a relaxing activity to fill your day with. But avoid anything NCLEX on NCLEX day, except well... the NCLEX itself.

Show Up Early

The last thing you want to do to do is fail your test by missing your appointment. Make sure that you know your way to your destination and arrive in enough time to use the restroom, drink some water, and sit down and relax. You don't want to be running around like a chicken with your head cut off trying to get to your testing appointment.

Go with Your Gut and Don't Doubt Yourself

I cannot tell you the number of times I thought to myself "It's supposed to be harder than this," while I was taking the NCLEX. I found myself in doubt of answers that I knew; I just had to stop and tell myself to stop doubting. If I knew the answer, then why would I try and tell myself I didn't? You have to be confident in your decisions on the test. Read all the answers and use critical thinking, but don't be afraid to go with your gut.

CAT : Computerized Adaptive Testing

The NCLEX uses computerized adaptive testing technology. What that basically means is that is choosing your next question based upon if you successfully answered a question. Once you answer a certain amount correct in a certain level you bump up to the next level. You then have to answer a certain amount correct to bump up again until you get to a minimum of 75 questions. Every question you answer makes the computer recalculate your probability of success. So based upon how many you get correct it predicts if giving you more questions will help you pass or not. So getting past 75 questions does not mean you fail the NCLEX, it actually means it's pretty sure you can pass it. However, it needs you to answer a few more questions correct before it can be sure.

Don't Psych Yourself Out Trying to Figure Out the CAT Process

Don't freak yourself out trying to figure out if the question you are answering is easier or harder than the one you just answered. In addition to the fact that you're just wasting time, and it doesn't make a difference, somewhere along the lines of 30 questions will be "test" question for use in future NCLEX exams. So you may be freaking out because you got an easy question after a serious of select all that apply and thinking that you bombed them, when in reality the computer is just throwing in a "test" question (that doesn't count) at random.

Most effective practice: have at least 2-4 headings

When you're writing your post, have your headings in mind first. It's harder to go back and add them after the post is done. Think about your main points, use the heading formatting built into WordPress, then fill in the rest.

Blogging Mistake #3 - Blogging for You and Not Your Audience

Remember, the focus is on filling a void within your niche and communicating your passion, which is based on a need. When you connect a need with a passion, staying focused on that message, the content you create will be valuable. People can sense when someone cares and has a heart to make things better. Conversely, people can also sense when the author has their own agenda, when they're not there to listen and engage with their community, but just to complete a transaction.

This is really important to consider as you grow and begin receiving offers for advertisements and other forms of sponsorship. If you wouldn't write about something without being paid you shouldn't write about it just because you are paid. It will come off as inauthentic and you risk damaging your relationship with your readers.

Most effective practice: keep your target audience in mind, speak directly to them, and address what's important to them.

What do they want to hear? What is a common struggle of this group? For example, Jon Haws over at NRSNG focuses on specific nursing school struggles, which is something we all can relate to! If you go to the blog on his site, the posts are categorized with the title, "What are you struggling with?". Readers know exactly where to go with their specific needs. As a former nursing student, he provides a sense of credibility and knows that audience well. By leveraging SEO, and knowing your audience backwards and forwards, you will be able to create content that will address many of the problems they are experiencing.

Blogging Mistake #4 - There Are No Images

A picture is worth 1000 words. Plain and simple: you must have at least one image. You should have a feature image for the post, with text on it that has the title of the post. The size of this image will likely be specific to your theme. If you don't have theme restrictions, you should optimize your image for Pinterest and make it 736x1106.

Images are essential to share on social media (we'll talk specifics in a later chapter). Images break up the text, give the reader something else to look at, and if leveraged appropriately, can really make the text come to life. If you want to get fancy, GIFs are also great at invoking whatever emotion you're trying to convey.

Most effective practice: always have a feature image, and 1-3 others if possible

We cannot begin to describe how important this is. However, do not head on over to Google and do an image search for what you want, save, and upload to your website. This is a huge no-no. You must have the rights to the pictures you post no matter what, but especially if you have the potential to make money off of the post. The only images you don't need the rights to are public domain images, those with certain creative commons licenses, and images you take yourself.

There are many free stock images resources, but use caution. Many of these free sources also require attribution within the content, which can clutter your posts. Many are also populated by users, meaning that anyone could upload anything. You may download it and use it assuming it is free to use, but actually be using someone's work. Certain image companies are notorious for pouncing on novice bloggers and intimidating them into paying hundreds and sometimes thousands of dollars for using images they didn't pay for.

Resources for free stock images:

- Pixabay
- Unsplash

It can be challenging to ensure images are legitimately ok to use and how to attribute them. Because of this, the $1-2 that many services charge for photos is usually well worth the investment. You can purchase stock images with licenses at any number of sites. We've listed a few below. More sources can be found on our resources page.

Resources for paid stock images:

- 123RF
- Deposit Photo

You can create beautiful feature images with text overlay yourself using free online tools like Canva and PicMonkey. Alternatively, you can find a freelancer on websites like Fiverr or Upwork to create images for your blog for around $7-20 each.

Blogging Mistake #5 - Copying and Pasting Someone Else's Work

We know this seems like an obvious one, but we only bring it up because people have taken our intellectual property before. People have taken blog posts, copied and pasted our work onto their site. We've seen people steal posts, and not even change the formatting so it was painfully obvious the content was taken.

This is one lesson from college writing that still holds firm in blogging: plagiarism, better known as copyright infringement in the online space, is not a victimless crime. It is theft. Not only is it inherently wrong, you run the risk of being sued.

Most effective practice: never, ever steal anyone else's intellectual property

If you'd like to use someone's work, message him or her for permission before posting. If you see that someone else has taken your content, message him or her privately and let them know in a professional manner that they must remove your intellectual property. Do not rant and rave all over social media and call them out. Privately message them, and move on. If they refuse to remove your property, you can file a DMCA takedown request with their host. If this does not resolve the issue, discuss it with a lawyer who has experience in copyright and intellectual property.

DMCA Takedown: "When content is removed from a website at the request of the owner of the content or the owner of the copyright of the content;[8]" and DMCA stands for The Digital Millennium Copyright Act.

Blogging Mistake # 6 - Your Posts are Cringe-Worthy, Not Share-Worthy

Have you ever read a post that made you cringe? Maybe they were talking about how ridiculous their manager was, or how weird someone's hair was, or made sexual comments. Or maybe they chose to ignore all spelling and grammatical considerations entirely. Uuuggghhhh… Cringe.

---

8 "What Is A DMCA Takedown? - DMCA.Com". *DMCA Protection & Takedown Services,* 2017, https://www.dmca.com/FAQ/What-is-a-DMCA-Takedown.

Most effective practice: get people to want to share your posts, not be embarrassed, frustrated or grossed out

The goal is to get people to engage with and share your posts. Why do people share things?

- They think their friends will find it valuable
- They think it's cool
- They think it's entertaining
- It communicates something they feel needs to be shared
- They connect with it; whether by identifying with it or if it brings good memories to mind

If you consider why people share thing as you're posting, this will help you increase engagement.

Blogging Mistake #7 - You Don't Have a Voice

When most people think about sitting down to write something, they feel as if they have to write in a very formal voice, like they're writing a paper for English class. Blogging is much more casual than a formal paper for school or writing an article for a journal. We've read blog posts where it sounds like a robot wrote it. It was nearly impossible to connect with the author.

Have you ever attended a speaking event, maybe a conference or a class, and the instructor just reads the words off of a Power Point? Ugh. Boring. You could have easily done that at home. Conversely, have you ever been to one where someone spoke with authority and personality, told stories, illustrated points, and connected the dots?

Which one made you want to consume more of that person's content?

It is the same situation with your blog. If you write like you're writing a hospital policy, people will tune out. Write content that is exciting, passionate, and fun to read; otherwise, your readers will get that glazed-over look on their face, and quickly leave your site.

Most effective practice: find your voice

Write with it. Record videos and podcasts with it. Be true to who you are and let that be evident in your content. Brands sell feelings, not products. What do you make people feel when they connect with you? Are you trying to motivate, comfort, or empower? What legacy do you want to leave?

It may take some time to develop your writing and speaking style, but try to find your voice as quickly as possible.

Blogging Mistake #8 - Spending Too Much Time Editing

If it took you two hours to write a post and three days to edit it, you're wasting time. We realize many people are perfectionists, but don't let that be your demise. You are writing a blog, not an article for the *American Journal of Nursing*. If there's an error here and there, it's not that big of a deal. Go back and correct it if you find it, but don't spend so much time editing that you never actually publish anything, or it slows you down so much that you rarely get something posted.

Perfectionism is crippling and has no place in blogging. You want to ensure that your content is ready for show time, but that doesn't mean it has to go through 12 rounds of editorial review. This isn't a textbook. It's a living breathing blog that can (and should) be edited as needed. Your content will evolve over time.

Most effective practice: write your post, read through it once. Go do something else, re-read it one more time with fresh eyes and either post at that time or schedule it and move on.

You may go back at a later time and find an error or two, just correct things if you see them and move on. Being too caught up in the details that don't really change the big picture can severely impact your time management. It's like the ICU nurse who cares more about changing the IV tubing when his or her patient is hypotensive. Yes, it's important to produce quality content, but the quality doesn't mean every single word and sentence has to be perfect; it's in the message you're communicating.

If you're super concerned about spelling and grammatical errors, there are things you can do. The first is to invest in a proofreading browser plugin called Grammarly. There is a free version available, but the paid version is definitely worth it. It helps review content, as you write it, and identifies more spelling and grammar issues than any of the free tools available. It also analyzes your language and offers suggestions to replace words you've used too frequently or changing voice for passive to active. Proofreading is also a task a virtual assistant can help with, once you start earning income.

Proofread, get most errors, and publish. Don't beat yourself up if there's a typo, and don't take it personally if someone points it out.

Blogging Mistake #9 - Responding to Every Single Comment

If you've enabled comments on your blog, your readers will have the ability to leave comments on posts. There are certainly pros and cons to enabling comments, including the risk of spam. Generally speaking, enabling comments is a good practice to build community.

If you have an engaged community, you will hopefully receive many comments. If you respond to every single one, it dominates the comment conversation of your audience. In his book, *Platform: Get Noticed in a Noisy World9*, Michael Hyatt compares this to a dinner party. Your content is your first course, but the conversation that ensues afterwards is the main course.

He states,

> "As the host, you don't have to respond to every comment. In fact, at a real dinner party, it would seem downright weird. It would draw too much attention to you. Instead, the party has to be about them - your guests." (Hyatt 195)

When looking at comments on a blog post, most view them to get the opinions of the other people who have read this post, not the original author. When someone brings up a good point, it's good to see the author respond, but if someone sees six different "Great post!" comments followed by the author thanking every single person, most are going to skip over the more in-depth comments that add to the conversation.

Most effective practice: respond to comments thoughtfully and only when valuable.

This number will vary for different people and websites. Michael Hyatt stated in that same book that he responded to about 20% of comments at that time, but acknowledged that number could fluctuate. His posts receive hundreds of comments. On your blog,

---

9 Hyatt, Michael S. Platform: Get Noticed In A Noisy World. 1st ed. Nashville, Tenn.: Thomas Nelson, 2012. Print.

allow people to mingle and discuss, and offer your response/ opinion PRN. If someone has a particularly mean or degrading comment, you may really want to respond to that to prevent conversation from going downhill.

Are you ready for hundreds of comments? Good. But don't be too disappointed if they don't come rolling in. The landscape of blogging has changed in the last few years and many of the conversations about your content are happening off your blog on different social media networks. If your posts don't blow up with comments, and someone asks a direct question, you should probably respond and not worry about the ratio of your comments to readers.

Having a good comment moderation policy is a must. In fact, many bloggers choose to review all comments before publishing to ensure they meet the standards they've set in place for their community. Even if you don't moderate before comments are posted, a comment moderation or community standards policy is helpful. If a comment is completely inappropriate, people are aware beforehand that you reserve the right to delete their comment.

Blogging Mistake #10 - Not Knowing When to Pivot

Not everything you do is going to work. You may try some post topics that really excite you, but your audience won't really care about them. You'll try a new way to post things to a social media platform that doesn't get much engagement. You can take the same content, tweak it slightly, and see engagement skyrocket. Try things; see what works and what doesn't. Being a successful blogger means you'll learn about a lot of things that don't work, and a few things that do.

Most effective practice: fail fast, know when to pivot, capitalize on successes

Wasting time on strategies that don't bring value, traffic, or revenue helps no one. Make sure your blogging goals are clear and that you only institute strategies that help you meet them. If they work, increase your efforts. If they don't work, dump them.

Do not be so in love with various ideas or methods that it clouds your ability to see the need to pivot. The priority is your audience's needs. If you're blinded by what you think is best - not what they're showing you they need - you'll be spinning your wheels. Like nurses have to stay on their toes and be able to re-prioritize in an instant as patient conditions and needs change, so does the nurse entrepreneur.

Blogging Mistake #11 - You Don't Have a Disclaimer

This isn't something we would include for all types of blogs, however if you are a nurse and talking about nurse-related topics, we highly recommend a disclaimer page. You never know what may happen in the future and how someone may apply your information.

Most effective practice: have a disclaimer page

Here are some of the disclaimers we recommend including:

- HIPAA
- Giveaway disclaimer
- Affiliate disclaimer
- Privacy policy
- General disclaimer
    - "These are my personal views and do not reflect the views of the author's current or former employers"

If you'd like to check out our disclaimers, go to freshrn.com/disclaimers and thenerdynurse.com/disclaimer.

Blogging Mistake #12 - You Don't Disclose Your Relationships

If one of your goals is to blog for profit, you're likely going to partner with many different sponsors and advertisers. Transparency in these relationships is a must. Your readers must clearly understand whether an article has been sponsored or if you use affiliate links in your content.

Disclosing your relationships is critical to maintaining the trust of your audience. It's also a requirement of the FTC Endorsement Guidelines[10]. Whether you've received payment in the form of a check or products, this must be disclosed.

---

10 "The FTC'S Endorsement Guides: What People Are Asking | Federal Trade Commission". *Ftc.gov*. N.p., 2017. Web. 23 Mar. 2017.

Most effective practice: disclose your sponsored and affiliate content

Disclosures are simple. The basic rule is that you need to disclose your relationship prior to the first link within the post. Also, Google guidelines require that you "nofollow" any links to the brand in a post where money has changed hands. Backlinks are valuable and paying for them can falsely increase page rank.

- **Nofollow:** An attribute you can assign to a URL to tell Google and other search engines to not count this link when determining search ranking. In short, it makes sure your link doesn't impact where that page appears in Google search results.
  - ◆ This is accomplished by adding rel="nofollow"
  - ◆ Example: <a href="http://www.google.com/" rel="nofollow">Google</a>
- **Dofollow:** An attribute assigned to a URL that tells Google and other search engines that the link can, and should, be used to influence search results. This is the default, and typically not needed, but may be the case if you have installed a plugin that makes all external links nofollow.
  - ◆ This is accomplished by adding rel="dofollow"
  - ◆ Example: <a href="http://www.google.com/" rel="dofollow">Google</a>
- **Backlink:** A link back to your website from an external source. These links may be dofollow or nofollow, depending on the source of the link.
  - ◆ For example, social sites generally give nofollow links while guest blogging generally nets dofollow links.
- **Page rank:** How high a specific page or post will appear when someone Google's a certain term. The higher the better.

You can insert a blanket affiliate disclosure at the beginning of all your posts staying "This post may contain affiliate links" or deliberately add something custom to each post as you add affiliate links. For sponsored posts, opening with "I've partnered with ABC Brand on this content" is sufficient. Just make sure your partnerships are clear.

Blogging Mistake #13 - You Don't Have a Call to Action

Again, your focus should be creating community around your passion. Therefore, whenever you're writing, you want to increase that sense of community and conversation. A really good post is a conversation starter. There may be some posts that don't really require an engaging question at the end, but most will.

Call to actions aren't always questions. Sometimes you'll have supplemental content available from an opt-in, a product or service you've recommended, or another piece of content that aligns with the post.

Most effective practice: include a specific call to action with every post

When someone has taken the time to read your entire post, they are invested. They are looking for next steps. Give them something to do.

Start the conversation with your post, allow people to comment and converse, and intermittently add your thoughts when necessary. Have them download your free offer or buy a related product.

Blogging Mistake #14 - Copying Your Own Blog Post Onto Different Sites

Copying and pasting blog posts, even if it is your intellectual property, is considered bad blogging practice. It's not illegal by any means, but it's just not good practice.

Duplicate content is frowned upon and you can actually drop in searches because of this. Search engines don't know which version(s) to include/exclude from their indices. They don't know whether to direct the link metrics (trust, authority, anchor text, link juice, and so forth) to one page, or keep it separated between multiple versions. They also don't know which version(s) is the authority to rank for query results, so search rankings will suffer.

Basically, it's bad for SEO and could render a duplicate content penalty from Google.

However, at the end of the day it is your intellectual property and you can do with it what you please. Just know neither of us could, in good conscience, advise you to do this on any platform. We don't advise on Linkedin, Medium, or Tumblr. If a company asks to do this with your content, say "No."

Most effective practice: do not copy and paste posts, and do not let others do this to your work

If you have a great post you want in multiple locations, then re-write it a bit to make it different. Be very weary of companies offering to "curate" your posts to their site and make it seem like it's a good idea. This most likely is not in your best interest, and if they are a larger or established company, chances are they know exactly what they're doing and really hoping you don't.

CHAPTER 6

ENSURING YOUR
CONTENT IS SEEN

"If a patient hits the call bell and no one is at the nurse's station, did it really make a sound?"

- Unknown, RN

Writing amazing content isn't enough to be a successful blogger. In addition to learning how to navigate the backend of WordPress, you must understand how to get people to your blog so they can actually read the content. There are many ways to attract readers to your site. The methods we will focus on include social media, search engine optimization (SEO), and email marketing.

Owning a blog is like investing in real estate. Each blog post you write and put out into the world is like a new property you acquire. The amount of time, energy, and effort you put into the post is ultimately going to determine that posts value. If you put enough energy in the beginning to ensure you've written a great post and are attracting the right traffic, that post will continually provide value to you and your audience. Each new post you write grows the value and ultimately your income stream. Buy a crappy house in the wrong side of town and you won't see the same profits as you would have if you had spent more time and money on a fixer upper in a great neighborhood.

In case you were wondering, yes that was a Joanna Gaines reference. Now THERE is an influencer!

The same holds true for every post you write. Each post is an opportunity to grow your traffic and your business. Take each one seriously and put the work in.

Social Media

One of the fastest ways to get people to your blog is through social media. You can start a blog today, write a post, and share it to your personal followers to see dozens and maybe even hundreds of visitors to your site in a few short hours. Social media is that powerful. Unless you've been living under a rock, you likely already have personal profiles on multiple social networks. Each one is a potential path to traffic.

Sharing your blog content to friends and family on your personal social networks is a strategy that is only effective in the short term. Your aunt may read your blog to support you, but typically she isn't your ideal reader. For this reason, you'll want to create social media accounts that are specific to your blog and business. For Facebook, this means a business page, for Twitter a new account with your blog name, and a new account for Pinterest. Depending on whether you've decided to build your blog as a personal brand or a business brand these can sometimes be combined.

When combining business and pleasure, you have to consider the consequences. If you share an article from your blog on your personal Facebook page one day and then next day an image showing your epic keg stand skills, you're not doing your blog or brand any favors.

As of 2015, social media controls 31% of all website traffic (DeMers)[11]. That was an increase of 9% from the year before. Ignoring social media as you build your blog and brand means you'd be leaving traffic and income on the table.

In Chapter 8, we'll provide more specific information around social media including how each social network should be used. We are sorry to say that auto-scheduling the same 140-character message

---

11 DeMers, Jayson. "Social Media Now Drives 31% Of All Referral Traffic". *Forbes.com.* N.p., 2015. Web. 23 Mar. 2017.

across all of your social networks will not yield the best results. Each network fulfills a different need and you need to use it accordingly.

In general, Facebook and Pinterest are the biggest traffic generators on social media. Twitter comes in at number three, but there is a huge gap between it and the leaders. Traffic from Facebook accounts for roughly 25% of all social traffic[12] (Wong).

Creating engaging and amazing content to get your content noticed on social media is an effective strategy to gain traffic. The work of social media is no small effort, with each tweet or status update taking time to compose and schedule. There are many tools you can use to help streamline this process, but none will remove the need for creativity and thought.

Once your blog has been established, social media is an area that many contract out to a virtual assistant (VA) or social media marketing manager. When making the decision to do this, you need to ensure that the person managing your social media understands your brand and audience. They must speak English as fluently as a native speaker and understand how each social network needs to be addressed. We'll dig further into social media in Chapter 8, but for now just know it's going to be a vital component of your overall traffic strategy.

Search Engine Optimization (SEO)

More than 6,586,013,574 internet searches are made every day[13] (Clark).

When we talk about search and SEO, it's impossible not to talk about Google. The term Google is synonymous with search. Throughout this chapter, you'll see that we use these terms interchangeably. Google represents the majority of searches performed, 75% of those searches, to be exact[14] (Schwartz).

One of the biggest mistakes that bloggers make in the beginning of their blogging journey ignoring Search Engine Optimization (SEO). When you decided to start a blog, you likely did so because want to write about your passions and by doing so, help other people. In fact, if you started a blog for any other reason you're going to

12 Wong, Danny. "Report: Social Media Drove 31.24% Of Overall Visits To Sites". *The Shareaholic Content Marketing Blog*. N.p., 2017. Web. 23 Mar. 2017.

13 Clark, Alexander. "Search Engine Statistics". *Smart Insights*. N.p., 2017. Web. 23 Mar. 2017

14 Schwartz, Eli. "Is Google's Search Market Share Actually Dropping?". *Search Engine Land*. N.p., 2015. Web. 23 Mar. 2017.

find it to be difficult. Blogging is a great way to earn an income, but if your primary goal isn't to share your passions and help others, you're going to fail.

Search Engine Optimization (SEO): The art of and science of writing content in such a way that search engines rank your content higher in SERP, and readers find your highly valuable content when looking to solve their specific problem, related to your keywords.

Search Engine Results Page (SERP): Used interchangeably with page rank. This is the ranking a specific page has for a specific search term.

If you start a blog based on passion, you'll likely write emotional and impactful content. However, if you neglect to ensure that the content is written in such a way that the subject matter is clear the content will not get served up in Google. Consequently, it won't get viewed as often or help as many people as it possibly could. Let's go back to the book example. If you wrote the greatest book in the entire world, but you put it in a drawer, locked it up and walked away, no one would ever read it. No one would know the value that book could bring the world. Your effort would be wasted. The problems your book could solve would still exist. It's basically as if you never wrote the book at all.

The same concept holds true when you write a blog post. If you don't ensure that it can be easily found, it might as well not exist. What's the point in writing something amazing if no one ever reads it?

This is the question you should ask yourself every time you write a blog post. Think, "If I write this and no one reads it, what value is it really bringing?" You can spend all the time in the world sharing your post on social media, and you may get plenty of traffic, but ultimately, they may or may not be interested in your message and the problems you aim to solve. All forms of traffic are not created equal.

The best traffic almost always comes from search engines like Google, Bing, or Yahoo. When someone searches for a keyword and finds your content through Google, they are likely to be more interested in the result it brings than any random person on social media. When someone uses Google, they're typically looking to solve a problem or answer a question. They want a solution to something specific, immediately. On social media, people are often looking to connect with someone or waste time doing something mindless. They're less concerned with the problems you can help them solve. Your content may spark their interest on Facebook, but it's hit or miss whether they actually need the information you are sharing.

Traffic from social media is certainly valuable. It's one of the best ways that you can build a community and one of the highest referrers of traffic overall. However, traffic from Google is the best way to find your ideal audience, growing your revenue, and your business overall. Why is this?

One word: Conversions.

Focusing on Conversions

When you're blogging for profit, you're going to have to have some mechanism of generating revenue. We'll dig into what those might be later, but for now just know that when people come to your site you'll want to think of them as customers with a clear action that you want them to perform on any piece of content. If you've written a great post about cardiac rhythms, you may include a free download of an ECG cheat sheet. If you're smart, you'll ask people to give you their email before you give them the download. The act of a person opting-in and downloading is a conversion. You've made an offer, they accepted, and convert to a customer, or in this case, an email subscriber.

Conversions are your bread and butter. Whether you want someone to click on another blog post, opt-in to an email offer, click on an ad, or buy a product you recommend, every piece of content you write should have a have a goal or something that you are trying to convert.

Not all traffic is created equal, you see. Some traffic converts at a rate higher than others. This will vary based on the niche and specific type of blog or business you have, but know that it's better to have a small group of highly targeted visitors that are more likely to convert than thousands of visitors that stay on your site for less than a minute and leave without ever doing anything.

Traffic from Google converts. You'll earn more revenue and get more opt-ins from blog visitors referred by search engines. The reason is simple, really. These visitors will often benefit more from the content that you produce because they were looking for it specifically. They will often buy more products and generally stay on your site longer. These are the visitors you really want to find you.

Another thing to consider is that search engine optimization is generally a more effective use of your time. Blogging helps you produce passive income, but every second you spend on a task takes away from that passive aspect. Anything you can set and forget increases your profitability and the time you can spend with your family.

As we've already mentioned, social media helps you build a community. This is incredibly valuable, and certainly should not be ignored. However, it is labor intensive and requires ongoing effort including daily tweets, status updates, and interactions. You can't avoid this aspect of blogging, but focusing on SEO can help you augment and increase those efforts.

The most efficient way to get people to your site is SEO. Google, and other search engines, are the best way to get free and targeted traffic to your blog. By focusing on SEO, you can write a piece of content today that will continue to send you a steady stream of traffic regardless of whether you send the first tweet about it. If you've optimized that piece of content to convert, you've created a passive income stream. Do this every time, hundreds of times, and you have a profitable business.

Passive income stream: An income stream that will consistently pay out with little or no added work. Rental properties are a great example of passive income.

It might be interesting that we focus on getting traffic from social and search with a different level of effort. Brittney spends more time focusing on search while Kati draws people in with powerful and engaging social media. Both tactics should be utilized for the most optimal blog performance.

What is SEO?

So now that you understand the value of SEO, you need to know what it is and how to actually do it. The concept of SEO is actually quite simple. When you optimize content for search, you write content and such a way that Google is well-informed of the topic of that piece of content. For example, if you want to write a piece of content about a "nurse resume" you'll want to ensure that you've written the words "nurse resume" in your content. It's a tad bit more complex than that, but that's the general concept. SEO is about making sure that your content is written in such a way that a human and Google can easily determine what your content is about.

When many people think of blogging, they think of it as a philosophical diary or journaling experience. You might think of blogging as just writing things free form because it's meant to be more emotional and personal. If the goal of your blog is just to share your own personal emotion, and you don't have any intention for anyone else to read it, then free-write your heart out. However, if you're reading this book chances are you want to use your blog to grow your business or impact the world of nursing on a larger scale. If that is the case, you need to ensure that the content you write serves a specific purpose around a specific topic and that a human being and Google can easily tell what that is.

It's not enough just to include your topic once, hidden somewhere in the body of your post. You have to be more deliberate about it. But before we get into ensuring a post can be recognized for the correct subject matter, you'll want to determine whether or not that subject matter is even worth writing about. Before you put fingers to keys, you want to know that people are attempting to solve the problems you can help them solve and that they are searching for the keywords you wish to optimize.

Keyword: The word or phrase your content is about. Ideally, your keywords are highly searched with low competition.

Also, note the term *keyword* can refer to a single word or phrase. It's almost impossible to rank for a single word in Google. Typically, keywords will be strings of two to five words. Every page or posts on your blog stands on its own in terms of SEO. Meaning, each post will be optimized for a different keyword. You can also have secondary keywords that you optimize for posts, but you will likely not be able to do all the standard on-page SEO.

How to Optimize Content for Search

Step 1: Find What People Are Searching For

The most critical components of search engine optimization and the one most often overlooked is keyword research. As referenced above, you want to ensure that you're writing content that people are looking for. You want to ensure that you're solving problems that need to be solved. It is simply not enough to write great content, if no one is interested in reading it. You can optimize your content perfectly, but if no one searches for that term, it will not matter.

Finding keywords to optimize your content for can be accomplished in a few different ways. One of the most simple and cost-effective keyword research tools is Google AdWords' Keyword Planner. By creating a free Google AdWords account, you can search terms that you are interested in learning what the search volume looks like. Google will give you lots of information about different terms related to the search term that you look for. This includes the competition level among advertisers, which often equates to how difficult it will be to rank for that particular term.

To get started, use Google Keyword Planner and select "search for new keywords using phrase, website, or category." You can enter a term to be presented with the average monthly searches, competition, and suggested bid.

This example shows results using the word "nurse".

Keyword (by relevance)	Avg. monthly searches ?	Competition ?	Suggested bid ?
rn	10K – 100K	Low	$7.97
nurse practitioner	100K – 1M	Medium	$15.18
rn nurse	1K – 10K	Low	$8.74
pediatric nurse	10K – 100K	Low	$8.50

Since Keyword Planner's primary purpose is to help advertisers determine which keywords they will be against for CPC ads, it shows information about the suggested bid around these terms. As a blogger, this information is invaluable. Average monthly searches provides a general idea of how many people search for that term.

Competition is related to the number of advertisers bidding on a term. There's also a close correlation to how saturated that term is in search. The suggested bid is what Google suggests an advertiser spend to get a click on that term.

CPC (cost per click): Cost advertisers pay every time an ad is clicked

CPM (cost per million impressions): Cost advertisers pay per 1,000 ad views

A good rule of thumb is to look for keywords with high search, low competition, and a high suggested bid. The number one search result in Google receives about 33% of the clicks for that term[15] (Sharp). If you pick a keyword with 300 monthly searches, and you rank number one for the term, you can estimate that roughly 100 of those searches will land on your page. (Amazing, isn't it?)

When searching for keywords to optimize, you want to find terms that have a decent amount of traffic but fairly low competition.

Wait, what? Competition?

Yes. The quest for the number one result in Google can be highly competitive. Many website owners and businesses spend a lot of time and energy to get their websites higher on the list of keywords they deem valuable. The amount of results for a keyword, the quality and age of a site, the quality of the content, and several other variables all impact how competitive each link is for a particular keyword. One of the first things you should do is search for your keyword on Google and see what pages appear. If every result is a big brand it might be a good indicator to look for another keyword that will be easier to rank for.

If you are using the Google Keyword Tool to search for keywords, note that the competition is a scale up 100%. So, a 1.0 is actually 100% competition. Anything with a 1.0 is incredibly competitive and will likely not be able to be ranked for. Finding keywords with a lower competition can be challenging, but worth the effort.

There's no set amount of traffic that makes a keyword perfect. Each time you do keyword research you need to think about the value of your content and your conversion goal. What that basically means

---

15 Sharp, Eric. "The First Page Of Google, By The Numbers". Protofuse.com. N.p., 2014. Web. 23 Mar. 2017.

is the keyword with less search maybe what you want to optimize for if it's more specific to your topic. This is especially the case when you're writing about content that will yield high conversions and profitability as long as the right people find it.

For example, if you are an affiliate for essential oils and want to write a piece of content around essential oils that can help relieve stress, simply focusing for the keyword "essential oils" would not be a good use of time and energy. Even if "essential oils" has a higher search volume and a lower competition than a term like "essential oils for stress management," the people who visit your page on that topic are less likely to buy products or services that you may offer. The will also generally get less value from your page. It's better to have 100 people visit your site every month that are really interested in exactly what you have to offer than a thousand people that got there because you were gaming the search engines.

Keyword research can involve a lot more information including domain authority and how big the sites are that are already ranking for the term. You can do the work manually by searching for each term in Google and using a browser plugin like MozBar. However, using a paid tool like Long Tail Platinum or Jaaxy can really streamline keyword research making the process faster and more straightforward.

Step 2: Write Great Content Including Your Keyword Throughout

Once you've identified your keyword, optimizing your post for it is actually fairly simple. Basically, you just have to include your keyword in a few key locations. This is called on-page SEO.

They are as follows:

1. The title of your post (H1)
2. Within the first paragraph, as close to the beginning as possible
3. In a Heading (H2) of your post
4. Three to five more times throughout your content, depending on length (bold the term at least once)
5. In the file name of any images
6. In the alt text of any images

In addition to ensuring that your keyword appears in the above locations, you need to format your content in a way that is pleasing to both readers and the Google bot. This means using multiple headings (H2, H3) to break up content. You should also include bulleted or numbered lists whenever applicable, images, and internal (links to your site) and external links (links to other sites) to relevant content. Making the content exciting and visually appealing helps readers consume your content more easily. No one enjoys reading a blog that is just a long wall of text.

Now that's a business nurse eye roll! … Anyone? No? Ok… moving on…

H1 (Heading 1): This will be your title and WordPress will create this automatically. Do not create an H1 within the content of your post.

H2 (Heading 2): These will be the main themes of your post. These break up content and describe the content found within.

H3 (Heading 3): This will further break up content in an H2 in lengthy posts or where it makes sense to further divide content.

Don't try to game Google by filling your post with your keyword more times than makes sense. This is called keyword stuffing and Google can easily identify it. Posts you do this for will rank lower in search and ultimately can flag your entire site for a Google penalty. This will drop all posts and pages from your sites off of Google search entirely.

Google loves longer content. At minimum, your post should be 300 words, but Goode rewards thorough and expanded content. "In fact, the average word count of a Google first page result is 1,890 words"[16] (Dean). This doesn't mean you should ramble on about a topic it if has no value, but it does mean that you should make an effort to write content worth consuming.

As you can imagine, it's much easier to optimize for search in newly created content. Attempting to update old posts with keywords can be difficult, since you're often changing the entire style and focus of a piece of content.

When you write content optimized for search you shouldn't sacrifice the reader's experience. If the language feels awkward

16 Dean, Brian. "We Analyzed 1 Million Google Search Results. Here's What We Learned About SEO". *Backlinko*. N.p., 2016. Web. 24 Mar. 2017.

just because you are trying to optimize for a certain term, don't push it. If you get people to your site, but the language is choppy and difficult to read they won't stay or convert.

Step 3: Get Backlinks

Google is like high school. The first result for any given term is the prom king for that term. You can be a fantastic person, but if you aren't popular and well known, you won't be voted prom king. The first result of Google works the same way. It requires votes, in the form of links, to appear high in the SERP.

Backlinks come in two forms: internal and external.

Internal backlinks are easy. These are created when you link to your own relevant content within the body of a blog post, ideally doing so using your keywords or a variation. It's a good idea to keep a running list of your blog posts, their target keyword, and perhaps a few keyword variants so you can easily have a menu to choose from when linking to your own content.

A good strategy to use to build internal backlinks to make an effort to include two or three links to your own content in every post that you write. Once you've published a new post, find three old pieces of content that are relevant and could benefit from including a contextual backlink to you newly created content. Add the link to your new content within each of these posts.

Internal backlinks are wonderful, but they will only take you so far. For some search terms, getting to the first spot in Google will require external backlinks. The higher the competition and the more people writing about this topic, the harder it will be to rank for any given term. Getting external backlinks is one of the hardest parts of blogging, if you do it completely organically.

In a perfect world, you would create amazing content and bloggers and website owners everywhere would be clamoring to link back to you. Your content alone would be enough to gain tons of backlinks to grow the authority of each piece of content. Unfortunately, this isn't always the case. Getting other bloggers to link back to you is tough. You have to hope they understand the value of including links to external relevant content and that they have written about content similar enough to yours to include your link.

The good news is that you can get a large portion of your content to rank without building any external backlinks. Finding low competition terms, good on-page SEO, and internal backlinks are enough to rank on the first page.

There are a few strategies you can utilize to get backlinks from external sites. Guest posting is one of the most effective strategies. Using this method, you agree to write great content, for free, on someone else's site. In guest posts, you can include a link to a piece of content you are trying to rank for. You'll also include a link to your main blog URL in a short bio at the end of your post. This is one of the best strategies to get backlinks to a specific page on your site.

Another strategy is creating highly valuable content and doing some email or social outreach to other bloggers that have similar audience who would benefit from this content. Infographics are a great example as they are highly shareable and, if they align with a blogger's niche, can provide a piece of content that is easily sharable for that blogger. This strategy is good, but you'll only get backlinks for this newly created content, which may or may not be a high-value post on your site.

Pro-tip: You may get requests from companies or businesses who are sharing with you an infographic, guest blog post, or piece of content they think will be a "perfect fit for your readers!" While occasionally, you may get something that's worth sharing, use your critical thinking skills to determine if it's a good fit to share on your blog. Your platform is valuable, so everyone who sends something to you shouldn't just get a free pass. Look into the content closely, the company, and decide if it's worth taking up a posting spot and place on your platform.

Creating an expert roundup is another excellent strategy. There are several ways to accomplish this. Some of the most popular include:

- Create a top 10 list of popular bloggers in a particular niche and email them once it is complete to let them know they've been featured

- Asking bloggers to provide a quote or tip around a specific topic and then emailing them once it's published

- Compiling resources on a topic that includes references and links to other sites and bloggers

Once you have completed any of these posts, you'll reach out to the site or blogger that you have featured and let them know about the content. You can directly ask that they link back to it and share it on their social media channels or just hope that they will compelled to do so without a direct ask.

Email Marketing

If you research the average amount of traffic sites receive from email or email marketing, you'll find the percentage to be low. According to HubSpot, it accounts for just 1-3% of traffic for their customers[17] (An). However, we've included it here in the traffic section because these are some of your most valuable readers. They trust you enough to provide you with their email address and invite you to send them targeted and specific marketing material directly to their inbox.

Brittney's Experience

One of the biggest mistakes I've made in blogging was not focusing on building an email list. At the time, I thought that I didn't have a product to sell so I didn't have need for a funnel or a list. I used services like FeedBurner or the integrated subscribe functionality in WordPress to send my readers email updates for my new content. This was all well and good at the time because I didn't have a schedule I was keeping to and the emails would come randomly.

When Facebook changed its algorithm, I realized that I was relying too much on social media to reach people who had expressed interest in my brand. Facebook posts went from reaching hundreds and thousands of people, to reaching a hundred (or less). My traffic from social media suffered and I didn't have a reliable way to communicate with an audience who had clearly expressed interest in hearing from me.

When you put all of your eggs in one basket, you risk losing everything when changes occur. Facebook could close its doors at any

---

17 An, Mimi. "Average Traffic Sources For Websites: Benchmarks From 15K HubSpot Customers". *Research.hubspot.com*. N.p., 2016. Web. 24 Mar. 2017.

time and you'd lose all the likes you worked to gain. You would lose access to that audience.

Email is different.

Email Lists are an Invitation

When someone subscribes to your email list, they invite you into their personal inbox. Whether or not they receive your message isn't regulated by a company attempting to increase their profit by forcing you to buy ads. Your email will always arrive. You reach every one of your email subscribers with every email you send.

Email puts you and your readers in control of what they see. You choose what to send them and they choose whether to open it or not. Facebook eliminates that choice and serves only the content it deems worthy.

The average email open rate for media and publishing is 22.14% with a 4.70% click through rate[18] (Chaffey). This means that for every 100 subscribers you have, you can expect 22 to open your email and five to click on content within that email.

Click Through Rate: describes the percentage of subscribers that click on a link within the body of an email. The higher the better.

Should You Automate Email Marketing?

You can use email marketing in a variety of ways to ensure your content is seen. One of the simplest ways is to set up an opt-in form with an automated RSS feed that will automatically email your subscribers every time you send a piece of new content. This process is easy and can help you get reliable readers for every piece of content.

This method works, but it's not the best use of your email list. If you haven't researched it, it may be surprising to learn that email lists are actually more expensive to maintain than many web hosts. There are services like MailChimp that will give you a free list up to

---

18 Chaffey, Dave. "Email Marketing Statistics 2016 Compilation". *Smart Insights*. N.p., 2016. Web. 24 Mar. 2017.

2000 subscribers. Once you get above that amount the prices start at $30, but also includes several automated features.

You want to ensure you're getting the most bang for your buck with your emails. This will likely mean taking the time to craft a custom email related to each new piece of content. You'll likely get much higher open rates, click-throughs, visitors, and ultimately profit.

There is a place for automation in your email list that makes complete sense for you and your subscribers: funnels.

Fun With Funnels that Aren't Cake

When you think of building an email list, you may think of one giant list that is a catch all for any type of email you want to send. In reality, you want to segment your subscribers by their unique interests. You want to know what those subscribers are interested in, what they've downloaded, and what types of products or services interest them. Simple mailing list providers like MailChimp complicate this requiring you to duplicate the same subscriber across different lists.

When building your list, you want to ensure you have a way to send the right people the right content. You also want to ensure that people have an attractive reason to actually give you their email address. Ultimately, to make blogging profitable, you also want to sell something to these subscribers. The process of providing value, capturing a lead/email address, and sending out targeted communications in hopes to convert that subscriber to revenue is called a funnel.

The basic setup of an automated funnel is:

1. Reader opts-in to list by requesting free download offer
2. Reader receives free offer and confirms subscription (making them a subscriber)
3. Subscriber receives a one-week email sequence introducing a low-cost paid offer
4. Subscriber buys low-cost paid offer and receives upsell to higher-cost offer
5. Subscriber buys high-cost offer and becomes loyal customer

If any at any point in the funnel your subscriber does not buy the product or service you are recommending, they are still valuable on your list. There may be a reason they didn't buy, which could include your email copy, their personal financial situation, or the perceived value of the offer. You can monitor your subscribers who convert to buyers to see your overall conversion rate. It's hard to pinpoint a good conversion rate for every type of funnel, but a lack of sales certainly suggests a problem and will require additional investigation to correct.

Once someone has opted-in to your list, you have the ability to send them any relevant offers and can repeat the funnel process with them. If the first product funnel isn't a good fit, send them an invitation to get another free opt-in that will add them to a new funnel and send them a new sequence of emails related to a different product and related buy-ups.

One thing you should never do is abuse your email list. When people give you their email address, they've invited you into their home. You are a guest. This doesn't mean you can flood their inboxes with any affiliate offer you come across or sell tons of paid advertisements to them. Taking actions like that will cause a mass of unsubscribes and could potentially get you in hot water with your email provider.

Finding a Great Email List Provider

There isn't one email list provider that is the perfect fit for everyone. If that were the case, there would only be one. Every blogger has different needs. Assessing this includes noting the varying levels of your readers' actions on their email and your site.

A basic email provider will allow you to collect email addresses, confirm them, send automated RSS emails, and may have some sequence functionality. Examples include MailChimp and Mad Mimi. These often lack the complexity to deliver downloads from opt-ins or tag the same subscriber multiple times. There are usually ways to work within these systems to provide similar functionality, but it may be cumbersome for your subscribers. You also may be forced to count the same person multiple times if you have them on multiple lists or sequences.

There are more complex email providers with more standard automations that are a tier above basic email providers. One such provider, ConvertKit, allows you to create as many opt-in forms as you want with built-in functionality to deliver offers and place subscribers in sequences or groups based on offers they download, links they click, or other actions they perform. ConvertKit, and other similar services, are generally more expensive than basic email providers, but when used correctly, can save time and lead to higher conversions and revenue.

Awesome Opt-In Offers

Getting people to opt-in to your list requires some effort on your part. While you may be able to provide exceptional blog content that will entice people to "subscribe for email updates," chances are that adding something to sweeten the pot will certainly help. You can create a small product such a short ebook, checklist, or video course and offer it for free in exchange for someone subscribing to your list. As described in the funnel process before, ideally you'll also want to follow that up with paid offers related to the free offer. Even if you don't follow up with an email sequence or funnel, creating the opt-in offer will increase your subscribers. This means you'll have a larger list of people to send content and futures pushes for products and services.

Opt-In Offers Ideas

- Ebook
- Report
- Checklist
- Email Course
- Video Course
- Discount Code

Finding the Best Opt-In Location

The location of your opt-in box or offer is a personal choice, but some locations will likely produce higher conversions. Popular locations to include:

- Top or bottom ribbon
- In the content or at end of the post
- Sidebar
- Pop-over or slide-in

Each location has advantages and you'll need to test different offers in different locations to see what yields the best results. Comparing different offers or different locations is called A/B testing. This can be done manually by simply changing the code for your opt-in and manually tracking results for a certain period of time. However, there are tools, such as Thrive Leads, that can make this process much easier by automatically tracking and comparing ultimately showcasing the form or location that delivers the best results.

Another benefit of Thrive Leads is the ability to create beautiful opt-in forms. While most mailing list providers provide an HTML opt-in form or a WordPress plugin, they are usually very basic. You want to create something eye-popping and really captivating so your opt-in offer will really make an impact.

CHAPTER 7

MONETIZATION

You've been working full time at the hospital and every day that you're not in scrubs, you're at home, working on your brand and content creation. As you've become more successful in your writing, you will receive more and more requests for reviews, guest posts, and other things that require your time. Now, you never have a day off. You're exhausted.

This started out as a hobby and cultivating your passion, and now you have real deadlines and expectations to meet. As you're learning more and perfecting your craft, you're really seeing how much time it requires to create a quality blog post, craft an image, publish it, and share it to all of your social media outlets. More and more websites are interested in guest posts and ways to collaborate. You're excited, but you're exhausted.

Sounds familiar?

Couple this struggle with the guilt about making money writing about nursing, and you've just described a large portion of the nurse blogging industry. There are so many talented online influencers that are either making no money, or barely enough to enable them to continue providing value.

Don't let that be you.

Many people are idealists and believe that nurses should provide free high-quality content out of the kindness and desires of their hearts. Financial gain from their content or image is an absurd thought to them. It would be wonderful if we could all feed our families and pay our mortgages with kindness and good intent, but the world simply doesn't work that way.

Blogging is hard work and there will come a time when you will need to be paid for it to continue to be worthwhile. The amount of time and personal financial investment required to create and distribute quality is remarkable. Because of this, blogging out of the kindness of our hearts is impractical in the short run and damaging in the long run. We all enjoy being nurses and taking care of patients, but it is a career; it is not a hobby. No one expects you to work a shift for free. Why is blogging any different?

As bloggers, we provide a service to nurses by providing tools and resources to help nurses better care for their patients. We should be compensated appropriately for not only our time, but our expertise as well. You should, too.

Our expertise, knowledge, and opinion as a nurse is valuable.

Your expertise, knowledge, and opinion as a nurse is valuable.

Do not sell yourself short.

However, it is important to draw the line at being appropriately compensated for your expertise, and manipulating people to earn money. If you are providing valuable expertise, and the time it requires you to do so prevents you from being able to work and earn money otherwise, you should be compensated.

There are many ways to monetize yourself and your brand, which in turn will enable you to be able to serve your audience better. There isn't a cookie-cutter, specific way to go about doing this. It's a good idea to try different methods and find a few that work best for you. Having a diversified income stream should always be your goal in monetizing. Don't put all of your eggs in one basket, because something could always change and that income stream would dry right up. First, we'll talk about our personal paths to monetization, as it's been somewhat different for both of us. Then we'll dive into different strategies you can use.

Monetization for FreshRN

I was writing for about a year before I ever made a dime. I was originally on a WordPress.com site, and enabled their ad services on it. I was compensated based on the number of hits on my site. I received $50 here and there, and then a few posts went viral and one month I received $1300. That blew my mind.

However, I ended up switching to a WordPress.org website to enable more options as far as formatting and advertising. It's been important to me to keep the site light on advertising because I personally hate going to a site where I have to weed through the ads to get to the content. I started getting more and more requests for freelance writing opportunities. At first I didn't charge because I wanted to get my name out there and didn't want to make waves and ask. I then started needing to request compensation because I simply didn't have time. I charged a few hundred dollars an article.

Then people wanted me to do product reviews or were sending me products to post about on my social media. I started doing that, and only accepting the free item and posting. However, I started to realize how valuable that was to these different brands to have an influencer posting about it, and more and more requests started coming in. I had to filter it somehow. So, I started charging for posts and reviews. People also wanted to send me guest blog articles to post on my site. I put a few up for free, but then again realized how valuable it was and was also being bombarded with requests. I started to charge for this as well, and only accepted the articles I thought kept in tone with the blog and didn't say yes to everyone (which was more difficult than I thought it would be!).

Around the same time, I independently published my first book. I did this both to make some income as well as provide a comprehensive resource to answer the same questions being asked over and over. Because I published independently, I just had to pay the upfront costs (roughly $400, although I wished I had spent closer to $700-$800), and then I received a monthly check for royalties from Amazon and BookBaby.

I entered into a few contracts with companies for endorsements and sponsorships, which offered either a lump sum compensation, quarterly, or after project completion (I learned a lot in this process, more later!). I also began booking speaking engagements, which provided a one-time payment.

I originally felt like I shouldn't charge for these, but it did require time to write, practice, and deliver the speech. I'm not able to work on other things at the same time, typically have to travel, and block that date. I've also come to realize that my expertise is valuable and needs to be considered as well.

I utilize affiliate marketing which provides additional revenue. I've also written three other books. However I went through a publisher and am only paid biannually; and the percentages for compensation are extremely low. Therefore, unless you sell millions, you're not making a livable wage off of a book published by a publisher.

I have just begun creating digital products. This has all evolved since 2014, and in May of 2015 I went from a full time bedside nurse to PRN status. I officially left the bedside in October 2016 because this income allowed it, I wanted to stay home with my daughter, and will begin graduate school shortly.

My income today comes from various sources: book sales, speaking events, review posts, freelance writing, sponsored guest posts, digital products, and affiliate sales. The amazing thing is that I have the ability to stay home at a point in my life in which that is important to my family and myself. The challenging aspect is that this income is unpredictable. Some months are minimal, and some months are much more profitable. My husband and I must be disciplined and diligent with our finances because we simply don't know how each month will play out.

However, as I have been able to devote more time to my brand, I've been able to create better and more meaningful content. Monetizing enabled this hobby to evolve into a career, and gave me the gift of time. Because I'm not in the midst of a work hangover from working 12-hour shifts the last four days in the neuro ICU, I'm able to really focus on what I'm creating, and researching ways to stay on top of my game.

When leveraged appropriately, monetizing your nurse brand has the ability to positively impact yourself and your niche audience profoundly.

Monetization for The Nerdy Nurse

I blogged my soul for years before I earned one red cent. During these years, I not only invested time, I was also investing money on website hosting, themes, social media, tools, graphics, and other related expenses. I had received many offers for sponsored content and other payments, but the guilt of earning money from my words always won in the end.

As my investments began to grow and my traffic began to increase, writing for free just started to get old. I came to terms with my guilt and got over it. I accepted my first sponsored post offer and never looked back.

Now, I have a strategic business plan for my blog and have my finger on the pulse of all my various monetization streams. I earn income from the following areas:

- Affiliate marketing
- Sponsored posts
- Freelance writing
- Ad sales
- Professional speaking
- Endorsements
- Consulting

When I first started accepting sponsored posts my fee was low. I'd sometimes work for $50-100 for a 500-word blog post. Each post would generally take four or more hours to edit and publish, not counting any additional social media promotion. I was only earning around $12-25 an hour, which was often less than I earned as a nurse on the floor. If you factor in the increased tax burden on self-employment income, I was earning even less.

I was thankful to have income at the time. As a relatively new nurse, with a new baby, home, and marriage, any extra income I could bring into my household was a welcome blessing. Early in nursing I was struggling to make ends meet. I had a staggering amount of student loans and worked in an area that pumped out nursing students. The hospitals kept the wages low and there were times when I wasn't sure how we would keep the lights on.

When I finally gave in and accepted payment for my first sponsored post, a switch in my brain turned on and I became a passive income machine. I looked at my blog as a business that could provide an impactful, supplemental income for my family. I started taking it much more seriously, investing in more tools and resources to improve my content, and looking for ways to incorporate additional income streams.

I've increased my fees for sponsored content as the traffic and value of my online space and influence have increased. I've also refined my strategy around them offering posts in packages with guaranteed social shares, reporting, customized images, email distribution and other bonuses. This helps increase the value to my sponsors and ensures the content will be seen.

Sponsored posts are great, but you typically get paid for these once even though they live on your site forever. While I have implemented a 12-month minimum on my sponsored post agreement, I prefer to invest my time and energy into content that earns money forever. My preferred method of monetization, and my biggest income stream, is affiliate marketing.

Different Methods of Monetizing

We've already talked about how a diversified income stream should be your goal. Because of this, it's important to try multiple monetization methods before picking a clear winner. There are so many ways you can earn income from your online presence. Over the next few pages we'll outline some of our favorites.

Affiliate Marketing

Affiliate marketing is one of the best ways to monetize an online platform. Just like the Ronco Rotisserie, you can set it and forget. Ok. Not entirely forget it, but you do most of the work up front and can earn income for years to come.

The closest comparison we can make to affiliate marketing is real estate. Each post you write is like a new property you acquired. You put affiliate links in the content that will drive sales and earn revenue. These are your rent checks. If you buy a house in a better part of town or invest more time and energy into making it great, you earn more money. Affiliate marketing is the same way. Your revenue is directly implicated by the quality of your keywords, the products you promote, and the work you put into it.

Affiliate marketing is truly a beautiful thing. Signing up for programs is easy. You can write your content in such a way that the affiliate links you include provide value and solve the problems of the readers. Affiliate links are also easy to set up. Simply link naturally throughout the content or include a an image and buy button with the affiliate link. Once it's done - it's done. Well, except for the promotion. If you're earning money from that post, you want to promote it forever.

So, what exactly is affiliate marketing? Basically, affiliate marketing is where an online retailer (like Amazon) has an agreement to pay a commission to someone (like you!) for sales. You basically work as a salesman for that product or service and are rewarded with a percentage of the cost of that product. You can totally do this and provide value without being sleazy or salesy.

For example, let's say one of us loves a specific stethoscope and want to post about it. Typically, when you talk about how great something is online, people appreciate it when you put a link so they can find out more and maybe purchase it. So, we write a whole blog post about how amazing this scope is and include that link for people to purchase it. If we are an affiliate with that company, we make the link to the product an "affiliate link" (a specific link to that product, identifying us as the person who referred this consumer to this specific product) so that when people click the link and purchase it, we get a small percentage of the sale, at no additional cost to the buyer.

It's kind of like a finder's fee, or referral bonus, for connecting the consumer with a product they would like or need. This does not change the final price of the item in any way. Companies under-stand how valuable affiliate marketing is because of social media and the power of influencers. Carefully selected influencers posting about their product are much more likely to convert to a sale than various ad space, and often much cheaper. This is the reason that many affiliate programs require an application process. Companies want to know who will be referring traffic and sales to them.

The major benefit to a brand with affiliate marketing is they don't just spend advertising dollars with the hope that it will convert into sales. They only pay commissions when a product sells. It's also great for the influencer because you are incentivized to sell more and your income potential has room for much more growth compared to the flat fees paid for sponsored content or the low rates for CPC or CPM advertising.

As we discussed earlier, transparency with affiliate marketing is key. It is important to identify that you are an affiliate with certain companies. It is so important in fact, that it's illegal to use affiliate links without a disclosure. Amazon has specific requirements for this disclosure, as do many other companies. Laws are always changing and evolving, however, currently you must have your disclosure within the post, before your first affiliate link. So, you can't have a blog post of 17 affiliate links, and then a small sentence at the end that says the post has affiliate links. You must put it <u>before</u> the links. As a safeguard/good practice, we both typically include a disclosure sentence at the top of the blog post stating, "This post contains affiliate links."

It is important to use affiliate links wisely. If you just go out and become an affiliate for as many companies as possible and just put link after link up, people start to think your only motivation is revenue. Be selective about what you'd like to promote, so people know when you're genuinely recommending something and not just doing it to make a sale.

Many companies offer products and services that can convert the nursing market. Some require just filling out some online forms, while others require approval. Some fellow nurse bloggers who are trying to get their course, product, or content out there may also offer this - so keep your eyes peeled!

You can also recruit affiliates for your product or service. If you've created a digital or physical product you can install a plugin or other tracking tool allow people to earn a commission when they sell your product. You'll ultimately sell more products. Thankfully this process is fairly easy as many of the affiliate plugins on the market automate sign up and link creation process. You'd simply set the rate, approve affiliate, provide marketing materials, collect payment, and write commission checks.

Affiliate rates vary by company and the types of products you promote. Physical merchandise is typically 4-15%, with some specific niche retailers going as high as 20%. Infoproducts (digital products) have a higher margin and are generally delivered automatically. This means the commissions are much higher to the tune of 30-60% with 40-50% being the industry standard.

Affiliate Programs

Some websites host their own affiliate program, while others go through an aggregator of sorts.

 Aggregator: A service that groups related content, programs, or tools in a single location.

On ShareaSale, for example, you can sign up to be an affiliate for thousands of brands. All affiliate programs will allow you to grab links to promote products. Most require you to apply to each brand/partner individually.

Examples:
- Amazon

- Zazzle
- Ebay
- ClickBank
- LinkShare
- ShareaSale
- Affiliate Window
- Commission Junction

Automated Affiliate Programs

If you don't want to sign up with each affiliate individually, you can use as special type aggregate affiliate sites that will automatically approve you for thousands of brands. They then provide javascript to convert any links on your site into affiliate links automatically. This is, of course, based on partnerships they have, but will likely convert a large portion of your links.

Examples:
- VigLink
- SkimLinks

Javascript: Computer language that creates actions on an object on a webpage. Often these actions occur on click.

Digital Products

Digital products are another great option. Just spend some time creating content, making it look nice, then package it up for easy download, and you've got a viable income stream. There's no packing, shipping, postage, storing, and other inconveniences that come with selling physical products. Digital products can be e-books (which are essentially just a PDF), courses, training programs, audio files, videos, and so forth. It is something digital you create and sell.

There are several ways you can go about this, but most methods automate distribution. Your success with your product really depends on market demand, pricing, and your ability to get it in front of the right buyers with the right marketing language.

You can also use an on-demand book printing service like CreateSpace, through Amazon, to get your e-book to print. This requires just a little bit of extra effort, but satisfies the audience that would really prefer to read a paper book.

Kati originally had the plan of making her first book (*Becoming Nursey*) just a simple e-book. However, she discovered on-demand printing and decided to do that as well. The customer places an order with Amazoh or another online bookseller, and they facilitate the entire transaction from receiving payment, to printing, and finally order fulfillment. The great thing is that all the logistics are handled by the pros and Kati gets a cut of the sale. The same is true for the e-book, minus the physical printing and shipping.

Digital products can be simple like one PDF e-book, or complex, like an entire course. The important thing to figure into a digital product is that it *must* be valuable. You cannot just pull something together that is just mediocre, charge for it, and then expect people to want to come back for more. Your digital products must not only have valuable content within them, but the person purchasing it must believe they have snagged a bargain.

Now, this doesn't mean your product has to be cheap. In fact, many spend hundreds of dollars for online products or services and still feel like they've gotten a steal because the product really delivered value.

A few examples of other nurse bloggers/entrepreneurs and their digital products (that aren't e-books):

- Elizabeth Scala and her annual Nurse's Week Virtual Conference, The Art of Nursing
- Jon Haws and the NRSNG Academy
- Renee Thompson and her online courses focused on nurse bullying

There are many options for digital products out there. We encourage you to check out different nurse bloggers and what they have to offer to get a better feel for what it all looks like.

Endorsements, Brand Ambassador, and Sponsorships

Because influencer marketing is hot right now, a lot of companies are interested in getting involved with bloggers and social media influencers. If you get emails that offer to pay you to partner with them, do your due diligence and get things in writing, preferably in the form of a fully executed contract. It would be prudent to have a contract in place before agreeing to take part a continued relationship, especially if you will be creating content about their company related produces and services. We highly recommend never adding a company to your website, social media posts or profiles without a contract in place.

These partnerships can be quite dynamic and differ widely, but let's dive into a few scenarios.

- *Blog sponsorship* - a company may want to provide a larger sum to sponsor your entire blog, which would entail their logo/company name in numerous areas on your site, within posts, and so forth

- *Post sponsorship* (native advertising) - a company may want to provide a smaller sum to sponsor a specific post, which would include a disclosure that it was in fact sponsored by them, and potentially their logo

- *Brand ambassador* - you would be a spokesperson for this particular brand and do things like post about them and tag them on social media, write blog posts, create videos and so forth

- *Podcast sponsorship* - in exchange for a shout out (length would need to be outlined) on the podcast, a company many provide a sum of money, typically based on number of downloads

- *Social media shares* – a company may purchase one or several social media shout outs. These are less costly than a blog post.

All sponsorships require disclosure, even social shares.

Each of these examples can be wonderful opportunities, or can turn into learning experiences. After being a part of many contracts, we both recommend ensuring a lawyer reviews a contract prior to signing, especially if the contract entails you creating original content or utilizing content you have already created. Please make sure this lawyer has experience with reviewing contracts and copyright.

We have also seen companies approach nurse entrepreneurs with the promise of "exposure" or "free" products, expecting the nurse to provide them with free content or shout outs on their social media. There are a few instances in which the exposure would be worth it, but that would be the exception and not the rule. If you are doing work, you should be compensated fairly. Companies may boast a large following and impressive stats on their conversion rates and hits. They may also tell you how things are "going to get really great for you, soon," but if they are not willing to compensate you for work, be weary of them. Remember, free products can seem nice in the beginning, but they don't pay bills.

We've asked our mortgage companies, and neither of them will accept payment in exposure or free nursing scrubs.

The common nurse saying of "practice with a questioning attitude" reigns especially true in these scenarios. Trust your nurse gut if you start to get a bad feeling about a company.

Pro-tip: Be wary of "free" content in the form of guest posts.

After you have established your blog you'll start receiving requests to guest post on your blog. Often, they'll even say "all I asked for in return is a link in my bio." These requests will often be accompanied by a generic compliment or a reference to a recent article you published. Don't let this get your guard down. This is merely an effort to get a free link on your blog from an SEO farm.

If you get these offers (from someone you do not know), send them your rates and let them know links will be nofollow and include disclosure. Sometimes they will agree. Sometimes not. Just don't let your blog be an easy hit for SEO predators.

Traditional Advertising and Ad Sales

A few years ago, traditional ads were hot. These are your banners, images, and text links that clearly appear to be an advertisement. A blogger could run a few Google AdSense ads and rake in a ton of money. Most advertising works by either using CPC (cost per click) or CPM (cost per thousand impressions). With CPC, you are paid whenever someone clicks on an ad. With CPM, you are paid per view. Sometimes CPC ads could earn as much as $150 for a single click!

But the internet has changed and consumers have grown increasingly more blind to traditional ads. This is one of the reasons why influencer marketing has been on the rise.

Traditional ads can still be a lucrative income stream. Companies like Google AdSense, Media.net, and even Amazon offer ad services that will pay you on a CPC or CPM basis. Simply sign up for the program and install the code provided.

When installing ads, it's important to pay attention to placement. If you put something in the bottom of your website, and no one ever scrolls that far, you will never earn any money from it. By placing ads in highly visible areas on your site you can increase your earning potential. However, you could also irritate your readers if there are too many ads or if they appear before content. Ad placement is a balancing act and you should test what is the most effective on your site.

You can also sell ads directly. An example of this is when someone wants to buy a sidebar link or image. You'll typically earn more by selling ads directly, but you then have to manage the ad. There are plugins and tools that can do this for you. However, for most companies a sponsored post is a better value and will yield more sales for them and repeat business for you.

Freelance Writing and Speaking

Once you start to really dive into writing and get quite a bit of content published, you may start to receive requests to write for other blogs or websites. While there are some occasions in which writing articles for free may be beneficial (like intentional link building for SEO), most of the time you should receive compensation. Writing a good piece of content requires both your time and your expertise - which are valuable. Do not sell yourself short!

Many companies have blogs, but they may not have the time or the expertise to write quality content to keep them updated. However, they do know the value of fresh material, so they outsource the writing to other people. They'll do a Google search for bloggers or influencers who fit the needs of their site and cold call/email. If they are related to healthcare or nursing in any way, that person could be you!

Rates for freelance writing varies based on your experience and expertise. If you're highly specialized or are "the expert" you can charge more. In general, a good starting price for a 400-600 word blog post, written by a nurse, that is new to freelancing is $150. After you have some experience as a freelancer under your belt, as well as more notoriety in the nursing industry, you can command $300-500 per post.

Quick Recommendations for Freelance Writing

- Create an invoice template for your business, email an invoice to them after the work has been completed (Wave-Apps is free and accepts credit cards)
- Negotiate a fair rate
  - You can also provide the option of discounts for bulk purchases
- If it's going to be an ongoing partnership, require a contract
- Specify if you will share the post on your social media platforms
  - If so, consider this in your compensation rate
- Specify if they get any edits/rewrites
  - They may come back and say they don't like something or would like something to be removed or added, make sure you limit how many times they can request this or else they could continually request
  - Up to two is standard and recommended
- Only provide freelance content for free if the circumstance is too good to pass up
  - This might include a post where you'll get a full byline, and in content links on a very large websites, professional nursing organizations, or another major group
  - This does include specific link building opportunities where you are promised "dofollow" links
- Never agree to be paid in "exposure" - you are doing work!

We both received many inquires related to freelance writing opportunities and have worked with a variety of companies. We both definitely waited too long to require compensation.

Professional Speaking

Speaking is another wonderful way to add to your brand, credibility, and resume. Speaking opportunities may be something that

presents itself later down the line. This will become m
you demonstrate that you are an authority within your

Initially, opportunities to speak will often not have any
payments. However, they will usually cover the cost of your travel,
meals, accommodations, and any conference attendance fees,
if applicable. This is one time where it's really ok to work for free, at
least in the beginning.

Speaking allows you to grow your network and build some of
the best brand exposure possible. It also allows you to travel and
explore the country, and sometimes the world, for free.

After you've established yourself as a thought leader, you'll want to
start asking for payment. For a one-hour speech you can expect to
receive $1,000-2,000 honorarium plus any related travel expenses.
Once you get to keynote status, you can command $5,000-25,000
for a talk. If keynote speaker is your goal, plan on putting years and
hundreds (if not thousands) of talks into getting yourself there.

CHAPTER 8

SOCIAL MEDIA
MUSTS AND BASICS

Trying to create an online business without social media is like trying to page a doctor without using a phone. Now we know there are paging services available that use text messaging and other fancy technologies, but ultimately you still have to talk to the doctor. Social media is an integral aspect of successful blogs. As the Borg from Star Trek would say, "Resistance is futile."

We have no apologies for that massively nerdy reference.

According to a recent study, customers who engage with brands on social media spend 20-40% more on their products[19] (Barry). They also exhibit more customer loyalty.

Even if you don't have a "product" it's important to engage with your readers/customers. In the beginning, you are the product. You want your readers to read more, increase engagement, and develop trust in your brand.

Your potential customers and readers are already on social media. They're online every day, sometimes every hour. They're already scrolling through to see what's going on with their friends, their favorite celebrities, the latest news, and get new information from the brands they love.

19 Barry, Chris. "Putting Social Media To Work". Bain.com. N.p., 2011. Web. 24 Mar. 2017

You want to be where your audience is. You don't want to be some blog sidebar ad they ignore, or a commercial during their favorite TV show that they're going to fast forward through anyway. You want to be seamlessly weaved into what they already enjoy. You want to be part of their routine.

Social media enables you to provide value to your audience that isn't all business, build relationships. and genuine connections. It also lets people get to know you. Your readers want to feel a connection with the person behind the blog. Even big businesses know this. That's why you so often see companies have specific personalities they use when marketing their services or connecting on social media. Blogs are meant to be personal and conversational. Social media lets you get even more casual so that your readers can truly get to know the person behind blogs and brands.

Your social media presence, regardless of the platform, should be about 80% play and 20% work. If you just share post after post of your own blog posts, people tune you out quickly. Remember, people go on social media for a connection. If you constantly push your own content, or a sales pitch, you're not providing that. You're talking *at* people, not *with* them.

Remember how we talked about *Jab, Jab, Jab, Right Hook,* earlier? Social media is the playground for this philosophy. You have to give 80% of the time through fun images, interesting articles, quotes, personal messages, and insight into your real life. Weave your pushes or asks in about every 5th post.

Also, ensure your asks are meaningful and elicit response. Posting a URL with a just the title is often not going to be enough to engage someone enough to click through to the article or comment. Social media is crowded and streams are full. Since you're only making an ask 20% of the time, it really has to pack a punch. Your right hook has to be a knock out, as GaryVee would say!

If you're just trying to get your content out there and not talking with, engaging with, and providing additional value outside of what you're trying to promote to your audience, you're going to fail. It's like calling a doctor about an issue and they just keep spouting out information and don't care at all about what the nurse has to say or needs. Isn't that the most frustrating feeling? Just like French frying when you should pizza, if you talk at people instead of with people, "You're gonna have a bad time."

People will unfollow.

People will unsubscribe.

They'll stop listening and engaging. Your traffic, brand, and business will suffer.

Building Relationships and Providing Value

We're going to dive into each social media channel and give you some tips and tricks for each one. Each social media platform has a different function. They're not all created equal. Each social network has a different purpose and you must engage your audience differently. A good post on Facebook looks different than a good post on Instagram or Twitter.

We know what you may be thinking - being active on your blog, and all the various social media platforms takes a lot of time. You're right. It absolutely does. But you don't have to have a flawless presence on every channel. You don't even need to have a presence on every channel. However, you do need to spend time and pay attention to the accounts you create.

Building relationships on social media is like building relationships with your patients. Think about that unsure patient who is apprehensive when preparing for a planned surgery. You and the rest of the clinical team all know how desperately important it is, but the patient isn't sure. How do you get them to see reason? How do you get them to agree to what you know will help them?

You build rapport. You invest time into them... get to know them. You ask them about what they think and the reason for their hesitancy. After they get to know you and understand your credibility and respect your knowledge, then they make their decision.

There are two really important things that must occur to gain the patient's confidence:

- You must have a quality product to sell (the surgery)
- You must provide value (the experience)

You don't want your patient to have an unnecessary surgery, much like you don't want you audience to think they've made a bad purchase. You want someone to trust you, believe in what you've made, and to be so happy with the decision they made that they keep following that they eagerly anticipating new content.

Don't be the surgeon who convinced a patient to get an unnecessary surgery that causes them grief and complaints for the rest of their lives.

The major difference in the nurse-patient relationship and the nurse blogger and reader relationship is that the nurse patient relationship is designed to end. The nurse blogger and reader relationship is designed to grow.

Tools of the Trade

Keeping your social media updated with fresh and fun content doesn't have to be daunting. There are many tools and apps you can use to schedule and automate content. This way you won't need to pick up your phone every hour and post something new and inspiring. You can have posts pre-scheduled and they'll go out automatically.

The work to craft great social content should not be discounted, even when scheduling ahead of time. It takes a little time and effort to craft great posts that will invite your audience to engage with your content. If you schedule your posts, you can ensure you have a full social media stream with content that looks great. You can then go back later and engage with your audience as they interact with the content.

Some great social media scheduling apps include:
- Post Planner
- Hootsuite
- Buffer
- Edgar
- Social Sprout
- Tailwind

There are many others, but these are the ones that we've tested and feel most confident to recommend. Prices for each of these services vary with some being $10 a month and others costing more than $50 a month. It's worth noting that you may want to consider using a combination of tools for best results.

Post Planner is a great tool for planning Twitter and Facebook posts, because it recommends posts that have done well on other pages. But you can't schedule a LinkedIn or Instagram post from this tool. You can schedule those on Hootsuite. Edgar is a great tool because you can build a database of tweets that you can reschedule automatically. While a great timesaver, it may irritate your audience to see the same posts again.

When utilizing these tools, make sure you take the time to make them appealing. This means using images when possible, creating an impactful message, and using links where appropriate. People click on things because they look or sound interesting; they don't just click on any old hyperlink.

Each social network plays by slightly different rules, in terms of what will be eye-catching. Ensure you have a good image, sized appropriate for each platform, with great copy.

Creating Great Copy

Copy is the text that goes along with your social updates or posts; it's essentially your caption. Clever, interesting, moving, thought provoking, funny, or entertaining captions/copy with a high quality photo are what get people to stop, like, comment, and share. Spend time on your copy; don't just write the first thing that comes to mind. Good copy gets someone to want to learn more - it's not clickbait. You want people to know what they're getting before they click on a link. You're not playing mystery date.

Clickbait: Is a post where the title or copy try to get someone to click on a link, out of curiosity, but won't end up providing value.

Example:

Title: "You Won't Believe What These Nurses Have to Do Every Day"

Copy: Can you believe what they have to do?

Point of the article: Nurses clean up poop and give bed baths

Creating good copy for social media is one of the most difficult aspects of managing your social media presence. Crafting a tweet requires you to consolidate your message and links into just 140 characters. You have to get creative and be concise.

There is an entire industry devoted to copywriting. There are people who do it for a living. There are books, courses, blogs, and tons of resources to devoted to crafting killer copy that converts. Don't get overwhelmed by all the "stuff" there is out there on the topic. With copyright, and really all things related to blogging and social media, we recommend that you find a few that you like and use those as your guides.

Sharing is Caring

The primary goal of social media should be to engage with your audience. Your secondary goal is to share your content and push traffic. Different social media platforms have different experiences (on Twitter you retweet, on Pinterest you pin, on Facebook you share), but the objective remains the same: you want your audience to like your post so much that they want to share it with their entire following. This multiplies your efforts and reaches a much larger audience than you could on your own. When a lot of people share your content, it can go viral.

For example, if Kati tweets something out, it will appear on the Twitter timeline of the 21,000 people that follow her. Let's say that just 10 of them decide to retweet (RT) her post. Each of those 10 people have varying numbers of followers:

1. 150
2. 2000
3. 6000
4. 1050
5. 500
6. 700
7. 4000
8. 720
9. 234
10. 972

This is a total of 16,326 people reached by these 10 retweets. This gives Kati's tweet a combined reach of over 37,326 people. This nearly doubled the size of Kati's audience, or impressions, for a single tweet.

Those additional 16,326 people may not already follow Kati. Sometimes one of them will see the retweet and think, "That's interesting! I'd like to hear more from that Kati chick. I'll go follow her." That's how you organically grow your network.

So, why do people share, retweet, or pin something? We share because we find it valuable and think our friends would find it just as valuable as we did. Maybe other people we know would benefit from a PDF database of nursing brain sheets, like the one that Jon at NRSNG created. We also share because we think it's funny (if I had a bedpan for every nurse joke I saw online...) or if it provides a sense of identity or nostalgia.

The field of nursing is proud; people love to talk and share about their profession. There is also so much nostalgia that comes with nursing because our field evolves so quickly. Talking about the days when every patient got a backrub before bed, when nurses didn't wear gloves, or when they used metal bedpans, really gets people talking! And finally, current events are also share-worthy, especially if you can connect them to your niche.

The Right Message for the Right Platform

We've already referenced the fact that not all social media is created equal. Posting the same canned response across all your social platforms will not yield the best results. That being said, there are a few rules that apply to all of these platforms:

1. Don't just post 10 things all at once, once a week and think that counts as being active on social media. People can tell when you are unloading content and trying to cram everything in at once. Also, this kills potential for engagement. It's kind of like talking to a group of people and people are taking turns adding to the conversation, and then one guy comes in all loud, says a bunch of stuff and doesn't listen to anyone, then leaves. Then two hours later, comes back and does the same thing. Nobody likes that guy. Don't be that guy.

2. You must have high-quality images.

3. People are not only interested in what you say, but they're also watching how you respond to others who comment and engage. Have you ever seen someone respond to something on social media that made you cringe? Did you comment to let them know it was cringe-worthy, or did you cringe, unfollow, and move on? Just because people

'en't telling you that you're making a fool out of yourself, 'esn't mean it's not happening. Good self-awareness and emotional intelligence essential on social media because everyone (and we do mean everyone) is watching.

4. Don't just start conversations, initiate them. Spark up an interesting conversation with someone in your niche. Go out in the world and find other conversations to comment and participate in. Leave comments on other blogs, reply to other blogger's Facebook posts, tweets, or Instagram post.

5. Do not just re-share or retweet other people's content over and over again. People are following you for your voice, not the echo of a collection of others. Share the relevant content of others, but keep it balanced.

Let's dig into each platform and discuss its purpose and how to maximize your reach and engagement.

Pinterest - "This is who I aspire to be"

Pinterest is a social network based entirely on images. It's also the social network with the biggest saturation of females. 81% of the 150 million+ Pinterest users are women[20] (Aslam). What a great place to be when your audience of nurses is about 91% female[21].

Pinterest is where people plan things. They plan weddings. They plan baby showers. They plan nursing school graduation parties. They capture images of things they want to learn, buy, or be.

When people go to Pinterest they are looking for inspiration. They scroll through the feed looking for color and engaging images that speak to them. If it catches their eye, they'll pin it to one of their boards or maybe even create a new board to pin it to.

Because of all the planning that is done with Pinterest, it's not surprising that this audience also spends money. Eighty seven percent of pinners are influenced by pins to make a purchase with an average order value of $50[22]. If you have a product or service, you want to get in front of this audience.

---

20 Aslam, Salmon. "Pinterest By The Numbers (2017): Stats, Demographics & Fun Facts". *Omnicoreagency.com*. N.p., 2017. Web. 25 Mar. 2017

21 "Nursing Statistics | Minority Nurse". *Minoritynurse.com*. N.p., 2013. Web. 25 Mar. 2017.

22 "Shopping Stats: People Pin In A Buying State-Of-Mind". *for Business*. N.p., 2015. Web. 25 Mar. 2017.

One of the great things about Pinterest, compared to other social networks, is that pins tend to have a lot more longevity. Something you pin today can be repinned for years to come. Pinterest is also a big search engine. This means SEO matters here. It also means that, in addition to seeing content in their feed, people can search for something specific. This is the reason that that pins have a lot more longevity than other social updates and can drive more traffic to your blog over time.

Creating a Pinterest Strategy

You should develop a content strategy and plan for Pinterest just as you would for your other social networks. This includes deciding what content you'll pin, and creating boards and corresponding descriptions. One thing to consider in this strategy is that Pinterest is the only social network where posting the same content multiple times is a non-issue. As long as you are posting to different, but relevant boards, you can pin the same things with the same description as much as you like.

Pinterest, like all other social networks, "Ain't all about just you." Utilize the 80/20 rule again here. Eighty percent of the content you pin should be images and content on other blogs but related to your niche. Having robust boards with a variety of beautiful images is the key to growing your account and utilizing Pinterest to push a steady stream of traffic to your site.

It's a good idea to invest in a Pinterest scheduling tool. Tailwind is the best available. It allows you to schedule your pins across multiple boards and chose an interval in between. You can post the same pin to five different boards over the course of five different days while online having to do the work only once. You can also group boards together. Therefore, if you pin a lot of resources for nursing students, you may have a group of boards around Nursing Study Tips, New Job Tips, and Nursing Mnemonics. One post could fit on all of them easily, and grouping together makes it easy to schedule things to all those boards at once.

It is recommended to implement A/B testing with pins to see what type of images and copy convert the best. You can easily do this by creating two images with the same post and sharing with the exactly same copy. Then post the same images with different copy. See which drives the most repins and click-throughs and post that one to all relevant boards.

Anatomy of a Great Pin

People often shy away from Pinterest because they feel it requires too much effort. Creating a great pin does require work, but the formula for a successful pin is actually fairly simple.

1. Find a great image that aligns with your message.
2. Buy it (Seriously. Don't steal images.).
3. Add the title to the image, or a related phrase.
4. Include your logo or branding at the bottom.
5. Write an engaging description that includes your keyword.

Pro-tip: When adding text to images, it's suggested that you choose colors that are already in your logo, align with the colors that are part of your logo or brand, or are present in that image.

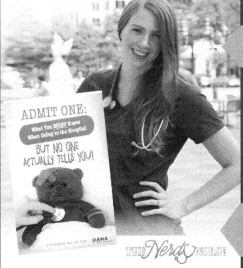

The Nerdy Nurse

Kati Kleber Shares Insight on Becoming a Nurse Author and Admit One

KATI KLEBER
FRESH**RN**
SHARES DETAILS ON
ADMIT ONE

ADMIT ONE:
What You MUST Know
When Going to the Hospital
BUT NO ONE
ACTUALLY TELLS YOU!

THE *Nerdy* NURSE

 Article from
The Nerdy Nurse   Read it

Get more Pins from The Nerdy Nurse

I recently talked to Fresh RN's Kati Kleber about her newest book, Admit One and what it takes to be a nurse author.

August 23, 2016

Comments

You saved to Nursing Pins from The Nerdy Nurse Nurse Nurse Eye Roll AKA Kati Kleber talks about her newest book Admit One and what it takes to be a nurse author. Admit One is the must-have book for any person admitted to the hospital. This is a great post for nurses, nursing students, patients and families.

Title:
optimized for search

Image Text:
Title (or close) on Image

Pin graphics:
Engaging and professional

Branding:
Logo on pin, standard color pallet

Rich Pins:
Verified account with rich pins

Description:
optimized for readers and search (keywords)

Bottom line: use Pinterest to showcase your content using beautiful images. Build robust boards filled with highly valuable content, complete with beautiful images. Optimize pins for search and conversion.

Facebook - "This is really me"

Facebook might as well be the entirety of the internet for a large portion of the population. Many people log onto Facebook for their news updates shared by friends, updates from loved ones, talk about what's going on in the world, and talk about their life. Content is somewhat curated (made to look nice), but also looks organic. People go to connect with the friends they already know, they're not looking to make new friends via Facebook.

Note - both of these definitions are as they relate to blogging and social media marketing

Curated: Content that is carefully selected and edited for optimal presentation

Organic: Content that is raw, unedited, and typically unsolicited. Also, content that is written without payment or appears in search results without payment.

On Facebook, by default, you have a personal profile/account. When you start a blog and begin building a brand, you should create a business page in addition to your personal profile. This helps separate content meant for different audiences. One of these audiences is your friends and family, and the other your readers. While there might be some overlap, these people are looking for different things from you. Your non-nursing friends on your personal profile are likely not interested in posts about your nursing blog. The audience on your business page don't want to see pictures of your kids naked in the bathtub.

It's not a good idea to ever post compromising pictures of your children online. There are some sick people out there who utilize those photos for horrendous purposes.

We highly, highly recommend - NO - we *insist* you create a separate business page from your personal profile. Attempting to use your personal Facebook profile and your business is a recipe for disaster. In addition, personal Facebook profiles cap friends at 5K whereas business pages allow for unlimited fans. Pages also provide lot of analytics tools and other capabilities not found on standard profiles.

Today, as we write this, you must have a personal account to create a business page; and there are different kinds of business pages. These options include:

- Local businesses or places
- Company, organization, or institution
- Brand or product
- Artist, band, or public figure
- Entertainment
- Cause or topic

Decide which best fits your needs and start a page. Have your branding match your website, and ideally have the same profile picture across all platforms. Create a cover photo in the appropriate size so that it is not blurry.

Facebook Terminology

- **Status update:** This can be a picture, video, or just text. It is uploaded to your profile and then Facebook utilizes their algorithm to determine which updates are shared to your audience's timeline

- **Timeline:** Located within in your profile or page, this is a list of status updates and shares that you have personally posted

- **Newsfeed:** Located in your homepage, this is a list of posts from friends, people, and pages you follow, which is constantly updated

- **Share:** Under every post is the option to share it, which would repost it to your profile or page. This is very valuable for brands because if their followers share one of the brand's posts, it reaches many more people

- **Like:** If someone enjoyed a post of yours, they communicate this by clicking "like" under the post. People are also able to "like" a business page as well, which means that whenever that page posts something new, it may be shared to your timeline. More likes are great because Facebook will view that content as engaging and will show it on more of your audience's timelines.

- **Comment/Reply:** Located below status updates, this allows your audience to engage and respond to the content of updates.

- **Follow:** If you are friends with someone, you are automatically "following" them, meaning whenever they post something new, it is likely to show up in your newsfeed.

  - **Pro-tip:** If you don't want to see what some of your friends post, you always have the option of "unfollowing" them, which tells Facebook to no longer pull their posts to your newsfeed. This does not notify them, but simply keeps their posts off of your newsfeed. This is particularly helpful during elections!

The Facebook algorithm, formerly referred to as EdgeRank, is the mechanism that Facebook uses to bring the cream of the crop to the top. Since the average Facebook user has the potential to receive more than 1500 posts, and Facebook only serves up around 300, there has to be a way to make sure that the best of the best are seen[23] (Walters). This often means that posts from friends and family will come first, and only highly engaging brand or business content will be served. Basically, by default your reach for each post you make will only be a single digit fraction of your fans. However, if they engage with it through comments, clicks, and shares, then Facebook sees that as a valuable piece of content and will serve it up to more people.

If you've got a great post with lots of engagement and reach, you can amplify those results by utilizing Facebook Ads. Ads can be very effective as long as the post is already performing well. You're able to target an audience to a very specific group of people. For example, if you have a post about something you think will be very helpful for nursing students, you can create an ad with a quality image, add a link to the blog post, and target it to people who are interested in nursing school, of certain ages, in certain areas of the country. This works great when you have a post including an affiliate product and you know it will convert if it's in front of the right audience. Generally, posts that have already done well organically will give you the most bang for your buck on ads. So, it's recommended to turn those into ads (or boosted posts), rather than creating one from scratch.

Things that work well on Facebook are short, high-quality videos with captions (85% of the 8 billion video views per day on Facebook are viewed without sound[24]), as well as blog posts with optimized images, good post titles, and good copy (Kirkpatrick).

With 68% of U.S. adults using Facebook, it's not surprising that the social network has a diverse and growing user base[25]. There are almost five times as many people in the 35-54 demographic on Facebook than the 13-17 age range. Chances are, the people who are liking, sharing, and commenting on your Facebook posts will be of this demographic, therefore it would be helpful to gear your content on this social platform towards them to get the most engagement for your efforts. In short, write content for the audience you are in front of.

23 Walters, Kendall. "The Facebook Algorithm: What You Need To Know To Boost Organic Reach". *Hootsuite Social Media Management*. N.p., 2016. Web. 25 Mar. 2017

24 Kirkpatrick, David. "Most Of Facebook's 8B Daily Video Views Happen Without Sound". *Marketing Dive*. N.p., 2016. Web. 25 Mar. 2017

25 "Facebook Remains The Most Popular Social Media Platform". *Pew Research Center: Internet, Science & Tech*. N.p., 2016. Web. 25 Mar. 2017.

Facebook Age Demographics (2014)[26]

Age Demographic	Number of Users	Percent of Users
13-17	9.8 million	5.4%
18-24	42 million	23.3%
25-34	44 million	24.4%
35-54	56 million	31.1%

Bottom line: have a separate business page and use Facebook to showcase your posts, share quality content from other bloggers in your niche, relevant news articles, create targeted ads, and have quality photos with good copy.

Instagram - "This is the ideal me"

Instagram is where people post highly curated content. People take photos, delete, re-take, crop, add filters and then finally post. Some people will delete them if they don't get enough likes in a certain amount of time! Instagram is where people showcase what they ideally want their life to look like. Therefore, you can't put blurry, low-quality photos on Instagram. People are expecting to see curated content that is beautiful. The more visually appealing your posts, the higher the perceived value.

Instagram Terminology

- **Feed:** The posts of people you've chosen to follow
- **Post:** The picture or video you've chosen to upload to your profile
- **Hashtag:** A word with a "#" in front of it like #nurse or #nursing-school. If you go to the search bar within the app and search various terms, every post with that corresponding hashtag in the caption or comments will come up.
- **Instastory:** A picture or video taken within the Instastory aspect of the app that does not post to your ever-lasting profile, but posts to your "Instastories" and is only able to be viewed for 24 hours.
- **Tags:** You can tag another person or brand in your posts by clicking on the "tag" option, searching and selecting the appropriate person/brand, then they are notified of this and it is part of their profile under the "tags" section

---

26 Apuzzo, Randy. "Social Media User Statistics & Age Demographics". *Jetscram, LLC*, 2014, http://jetscram.com/blog/industry-news/social-media-user-statistics-and-age-demographics-2014/.

Hashtags are important on Instagram. Whenever you post your high-quality picture, have a good caption with emojis, as well as hashtags. People will search hashtags (like #nurse #nursingschool #nursejobs and so forth) and then see all of the posts that have that particular hashtag. You want yours to show up, and therefore connect with people you wouldn't have connected with otherwise.

A good tip for optimizing your content with hashtags is to post a few key hashtags in your description with your initial post. Then add a comment with any additional hashtags you have. Your posts will still show up for those hashtags, but it makes your post look a lot cleaner.

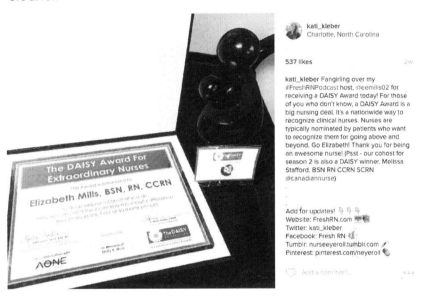

Example of an Instagram post with hashtags, emoticons, and tagging others

Unlike all other social platforms, you cannot add clickable links to each post.. Keep this in mind, because you can't just type out a long link like freshrn.com/nurse-bloggers9987239nfjdkjn and expect people to transcribe that into an internet browser. A work-around (nurses love work-arounds!) is to refer people to your blog for your latest post, and have your blog be the link in your bio. Clickable links are also available in post if you purchase advertising. Most people don't. So if you've ever seen someone post something and write, "Link in bio" at the end, that's why. They want to provide the reader with a fast and easy way to get to their content.

Pro-tip: Since you're only allowed 1 link in your bio, it's a great idea to use it to link to a highly converting opt-in offer. That way you can send those people more of you great content.

Facebook owns Instagram so they are interconnected. You can purchase ads on Facebook and have the option of having your ad also on Instagram.

Instastories is a new development within the platform. These are pictures that are not at all highly curated (in fact the more organic and real, the better) and provide a look into the behind the scenes of someone's life. The regular Instagram feed is like a magazine, perfected and polished. Instastories are like your home movies… raw, unedited, funny, honest. You take an "Instastory" and it's posted to a section of your profile, then the picture is only there for 24 hours. You have the capability to see how many people have viewed it, as well as the capability to save it. If you don't save it within the 24 hours, it's gone forever. You can use Instastories to show a behind the scenes look at video creation, blog writing, or notify of a blog post being published, or just a look into your life. People love behind-the-scenes peeks because it makes them feel important and like they're part of what you're creating. It makes people feel special and near the action, even if they're thousands of miles away.

Bottom line: use your Instagram feed to showcase your high-quality photos, use hashtags, and write good copy (catchy, funny, insightful, quotable, valuable), and use your Instastories to give followers a peek into a behind the scenes of both your personal and professional life.

Twitter - "These are my raw thoughts"

Twitter can be quite daunting, but it is an absolute must for bloggers and people looking to market themselves online. Remember how Facebook is where you connect with your friends and people you already know? Twitter is the opposite. Most people on Twitter don't personally know the people they regularly interact with on the platform.

To get started on Twitter, you create an account and begin to follow people, brands, businesses, or institutions that interest you. This could include politicians, universities, celebrities, scientists, authors, nurses, and people within your niche. Next you share short posts, sometimes referred to as micro-blogs.

Twitter is essentially the status update function of Facebook, except you are limited to 140 characters. You can include images, gifs, and links. Also remember that you're updating a bunch of people who like similar things as you, but you likely don't personally know. Therefore, updating people on your kids and frustrations over and over again probably won't net much engagement, but posting valuable content related to your niche will.

You're also able to respond to one another and retweet what other people say. A retweet is essential copying and pasting, or quoting, someone else's tweet (including their name) to your own timeline, so all of your followers get to see it. You can also reply or like tweets.

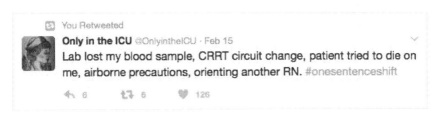

Example of a retweet: @Kati_Kleber retweeted @OnlyInTheICU

What you end up finding is people are much more honest about their opinions on Twitter because they're talking at and with likeminded people. Also, you can initiate conversations with people with whom you'd never speak to otherwise. You can follow CNO's of major health organizations, NYT best-selling authors, local news networks and authorities, and even your nurse idol! You can retweet them, comment on something they've said, and maybe they will follow you back eventually and start to see the great content and engagement you've got going on.

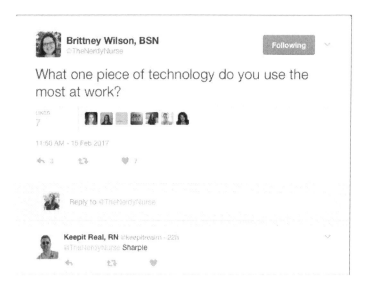

Example of a tweet and a response from someone else

The networking capabilities on Twitter are astounding. People land jobs because of Twitter. Seriously. Do not underestimate the power of this social platform.

Twitter is also the land of live events. "Live-tweeting" is when someone is tweeting as they are watching an event occur. People will live-tweet awards shows, premieres of highly-anticipated shows, presidential debates, major sporting events, conferences and educational events, and even during major events in our society (protests) and as well as disasters. During some of the mass shootings, when people were hiding in rooms they would tweet out about their safety or situation.

Twitter is also where the birth of the hashtag occurred. Just like on Instagram, hashtags are used to identify a tweet/post to similar content. If anyone ever searches or clicks on that hashtag, all tweets with that that hashtag will appear. This is helpful when you're looking to chat about a specific topic that may be particularly relevant to what you're doing. For example, if you wanted to write something on problems nursing students have, you could search #nursingstudentproblems.

Twitter is very now and in the moment. Like we said before, Pinterest is where content goes to live forever. Twitter is right here, right now. Just because you tweeted something at 0850 this am, doesn't mean everyone is going to see it. You may need to tweet it at different times during the day to reach more people. Although

Twitter doesn't filter out content, there's just no way humanly possible for any person to see all the tweets in their stream.

However, do not make the cardinal mistake of tweeting a confusing call to action. If you put a link to go to, a hashtag, and tag four other people your audience can't tell what you want them to do. They just skip engaging altogether and move on. Each tweet should have a clear result in mind. Concise, relatable, catchy, sharable tweets are the most engaging. Tweet something you want someone to like so much that they want to proudly share it with their followers.

Twitter Terminology

- **Handle:** Your username. Kati's handle is @Kati_Kleber and Brittney's is @TheNerdyNurse

- **Tweet:** A status update that can consist of text, a picture, gif image, poll, or link, but it is limited to 140 characters

- **Sponsored tweet:** A tweet that was paid to reach more people, and you'll know it's sponsored because it's labeled appropriately with #ad, #spon, or #af

- **Retweet:** Similar to the "share" option on Facebook, this enables you to tweet someone else's tweet to your page, all while keeping the original poster's information there (example below). You even have the option to add your own comment or information to the retweet by clicking "quote tweet"

- **Hashtag:** Twitter is where the hashtag was born. Hashtags basically group similar content together and make it easier to identify themes within content. They're also often used as punchlines in jokes. If you go to the search bar and search a hashtag, anything posted with that hashtag will come up

- **Live-tweeting:** Tweeting updates as they are happening

  - Events that are typically "Live-tweeted" are elections, major sporting events, award ceremonies, conferences, and concerts, to name a few

Bottom line: use Twitter to follow and connect with influencers in your niche, start and engage in conversations with people you don't know, use hashtags, share links (not just your content, but other helpful and relevant content), and don't just retweet everyone.

LinkedIn - The "professional" me

LinkedIn is the professional social media platform. Many people can take this platform for granted, but it's highly valuable for bloggers. Just like all social networks, it has its unique value and functionality.

If you're seeking traditional employment, LinkedIn is an absolute must. It is your professional image and acts as your professional resume. Roughly 80% of employers Google potential job candidates prior to their interview[27]. LinkedIn is one of the primary places they visit from these results. Use LinkedIn to craft how you want to be viewed in the professional world.

LinkedIn isn't just about getting work in the traditional sense. You can use LinkedIn to professionally network with other influencers. You can also use it as a way to capture verified testimonies of the quality of your work. If you're a freelancer or speaker, ask all of your clients to leave a testimonial on your LinkedIn page. You can then simply copy and paste this information to your testimonials page on your blog.

You can also use LinkedIn in a similar fashion to other social networks. There is a wall where you can share content that your connections can consume and engage with. You can even create a separate business page. In fact, the business page on LinkedIn is the only social channel where 100% of your content should be all about you and your brand.

In general, your content on LinkedIn should be much more professional than any other social network. Post your most polished and professional content and professional content from others here. Leave the memes, inspiring quotes, and funny commentary to other platforms. When you're on LinkedIn, mean business.

Bottom line: use LinkedIn to showcase your professional image to the world including a public version of your resume, links and images to your content and highly related professional content, and requesting and displaying testimonials for your services.

---

27 "What Do Over 80% Of Employers Do BEFORE Inviting You To An Interview? | CHE Career Exploration Center". *Blogs.cornell.edu.* N.p., 2014. Web. 25 Mar. 2017.

Social Media is a Must

There is absolutely no getting around it: you must use social media if you want your blog to be successful. At first, this seems like a very daunting task, especially if you only casually use social media today. You don't have to try to get thousands of followers overnight. Commit to learning something new each week and trying to get better and better at each platform. Also, we realize that it can be a little scary hopping on social media and putting yourself out there. The more comfortable and confident you are with yourself and your voice, the easier it will become.

CHAPTER 9

PRACTICAL
CONSIDERATIONS

C reating content and a social media following is one thing, but keeping your blog and business organized is another. In this chapter, we're going to take a dive into some of the more practical aspects essential to implement early on while you're building your business. From bookkeeping and branding, all the way to copyright protection. If you want to ensure that you're doing right by your business, this is your chapter.

Business Structure, Finances, and Brand Basics

Let's dig into some important general considerations, bookkeeping and financial aspects, as well as some basic brand needs. These are all big-picture aspects of the blogging business. While you could just put your head down, write content, and engage on social media, you won't be able to grow your blog into a business if you don't have the right foundation in place. You have to set goals and decide what you want out of your blog. If you don't have some the big picture, structure, and vision defined, you'll run around in circles and encounter a lot of headaches. These important organizational things are easier to implement while the business is smaller. They will make things run much smoother in the long run, especially as new opportunities present themselves at unpredictable times.

Business Structure and Tax Talk

When you are starting your business, forming a corporation to protect your personal assets is worth considering. While there are several business structures you could use, the most popular for blogs are Limited Liability Corporation (LLC) or an S Corporation (S Corp). If you intend to make money out of your blog, incorporating is something you should consider doing sooner rather than later. You can run a blog as a sole proprietor, and many people do. Just make sure you research all your options to see what makes the most sense for your unique situation.

This process creates an entirely different entity for your business, separate from yourself as an individual. Your personal assets are not at risk, should anything happen to the business itself. You get to accept checks in your business name, which looks much more professional. Also, depending on the opportunities and contracts coming your way, you may need to provide a social security or tax identification number to be able to obtain various tax forms at year-end.

Setting up an LLC is actually fairly simple in most states. Currently, in Tennessee and Georgia, the process is done entirely online. Search for the process in your state and simply follow the steps. If you need extra assistance, ask a business-savvy friend or look at some of the resources available on sites like LegalZoom.

The cost for incorporating varies by state. The rules of incorporating a business also vary by state. For example, in Georgia you can register as an LLC for $50 and your file taxes for your business as part of schedule C. You pay normal state, income, and self-employment tax based on your total household income and nothing extra based on business. However, in Tennessee an LLC is $300 and you also have to pay a minimum of 6.5% in franchise and excise tax on the income your business earns. However, since Tennessee has no state income tax, it works out about the same in the end.

There are also some tax and other rules that vary by the county you live in. These may be extra annual fees, the need for a business license, or other taxes. Before deciding any legal structure, which could potentially have a financial impact, but be sure to do your research about the specific rules, and pros and cons in your state.

If legal protection is the only reason you plan to incorporate or the tax burden of your state's incorporating rules make it impractical, you may consider maintaining your business as a sole proprietorship and just investing in some good liability insurance. Even when incorporated, having liability insurance is just a smart idea that could save you lots of money should you make a mistake and have potential legal trouble.

Whether you decide to incorporate or not, it's a good idea to register for a tax ID on the IRS website. Much of the income you earn on your blog will require you complete 1099s. It's not a good idea to just have your social security number floating around on these documents. You can use a tax ID instead. Registering for one is easy. If you have created a business structure you will select LLC (or whatever option you've chosen), if not you can register for one as a sole proprietor.

Finances

Because this is now your business, you need to keep your business finances separate from your personal finances. This is necessary for tax purposes. Blog income has different rules than W2 income and you need to be sure you know what is what. Also, most companies tend to prefer to write a check to another business. Therefore, it's prudent to open a business checking account at your bank. Other services your bank provides, such as online payments, can be helpful as well.

Payments may not always come in check form. In fact, many times the best way to request money is through online services. PayPal is the most popular service to do this, but other services such as Venmo can fulfill the same function. Ultimately, it's easier to have an integrated system where you build invoices, track expenses, receive payments, and track income in one place.

Bookkeeping is an essential aspect of your business. Whenever someone needs to pay you for something (like a speaking event, guest blog post, and so forth), you should issue them an invoice. There are free invoice services online, as well as templates available within Microsoft Word and other programs. Likewise, when someone requires payment from you, they should issue you an invoice for your bookkeeping. Paypal, Venmo, and so forth also have capabilities to submit invoices, and pay and receive payment within the service, making this process as fast and smooth as possible. Keep a record of your income and expenses by saving your receipts and invoices. Doing this as you go is a must, as attempting to collect this information at the end of the year will drive you batty.

There are many great online bookkeeping tools that really make maintaining the finances of a business a breeze. Services like Quick-

Books, FreshBooks, and Wave Apps all allow you to manage the finances of your business. Wave Apps is a great tool because it's free, but also has advanced features, like the ability to connect to your bank account to automatically add income and expenses. You can also generate invoices that accept card payments and automatically resend if they haven't been paid by the due date.

As your business grows, you may want to think about hiring a bookkeeper. If you begin earning a substantial amount, you also may need to look into paying quarterly taxes. Additionally, make sure you are planning for your annual taxes as well and considering the self-employment tax on your wages. Most contract work will not take out taxes and you will be responsible for paying that at the end of the year. Depending on how much you earn, you could owe a substantial amount in taxes, therefore you must plan appropriately and save at least 30% of blogging income until after your taxes for that year are paid.

Brand Basics

Your brand is your business' identity. Having a consistent professional face throughout your online presence and business contacts is essential. After you finalize a brand, logo, and tagline, there are a few things to get set up.

We've already established that self-hosted WordPress is the best route. So, you must purchase your domain name. This is critical. Nothing screams, "I'm not serious" like a web address with .weebly. com or .blogspot.com. The cost to purchase a domain name is small ($10-15 a year) and well worth the investment. Once you've secured your domain name, and set up your site with a host, you want to ensure that you can get an email address with your domain name in it. This is usually done at your website host, but can also be set up through a 3rd party service like Google Apps.

Basically, you want your emails to look professional and your business to look legitimate. Do that by creating an email on your domain. For example, instead of yourblogname@gmail.com, use something like jane.smith@yourblogname.com. This is a small, but powerful difference. Do not overlook this. Also, you should create a professional signature with your credentials and role in the business. Many people also put links to their social media accounts on their signature line as well.

Next, create some business cards including your contact information, URL, and logo. You never know when you run into someone who is a blogger, nurse, author, or someone within your industry with whom you'd like to network. It is helpful to be able to pull a professional business card from your wallet or bag to maintain those networking connections. This is a must at conferences!

Finally, considering trademarking your brand. This adds another level of protection to you, your business, and your intellectual property. This can be an expensive endeavor and may involve speaking with a trademark lawyer if you're not comfortable submitting the paperwork yourself. Therefore, this may come a while after you've actually started your business.

Contracts

If you begin to work with companies with whom you will have a long-term relationship, you're likely going to have a contract in place. In fact, many companies will have contracts in place for even a single sponsored post. The more regulations of an industry, the more likely a contract will be required. For example, insurance and financial companies will almost always require a contract.

While contracts are recommended for one-off deals, they are a must for long-term partnerships.

One-off: A single instance. One-off deals, posts, or work is usually a single blog post or a set number of social media shares without the expectation of long term or recurring work.

If you partner with a company to create content for a certain amount of time, you'll want to ensure you have a contract in place which clearly specifies the responsibilities of each party. Have a lawyer review the contract who is experienced with contracts of this nature. Some companies, particularly larger ones, will create a contract requiring you to agree to absurd terms like the ability to keep your content forever, to change it, or remove your name from it. A lawyer can review it, make suggestions for changes to make the contract more in your favor, and return it.

Kati's Biggest Contract Mistake

In a time of exhaustion and excitement over potential growth, I signed a contract with company in which I was not fully aware of what it entailed. Without realizing what I was doing at the time, this contract gave this company a perpetual license to edit and repurpose any and all of my original content/blog posts from my site, to theirs. What I thought was going to be 10 or less posts, ended up being 46; basically, almost an entire year of content. I was not checking back to see what was happening on the back end, as I trusted them. They have since removed my name from my original posts pulled to their site, so it looks like an anonymous editor from their team had all of these very personal experiences, but they were actually mine.

It is a red flag if the company is at all pushy while you are reviewing a contract. You should be granted enough time to appropriately review something you are agreeing to. The only exception to this is a single post on a tight timeline. You should still have the contract reviewed, but also charge a rush fee.

Guard your intellectual property with all of your might. Keep hard copies of all of your contacts on file.

Red flags on contracts include:

- The term "in perpetuity," which means never-ending.
- The ability to edit your work.
- Agreeing to arbitration, which means that if you needed litigation against them, you would go to a specific kind of court, which may not end in your favor.
- Agreeing to arbitration at an inconvenient location. The company may include a clause that states that if you wanted to take that company to court, you'd have to do so in their location. So, if you live in Maine and are signing a contract with a company in San Francisco, it would be considerably more expensive to hire a lawyer in California than a local one in Maine.
- Non-compete clauses that are vague and impossible to maintain.
- Non-disclosures that would be impossible to maintain.

Consider contracts carefully. We recommend utilizing a lawyer to review them, especially if it encompasses a lot of work or is in a new area. Furthermore, some companies will include ridiculous clauses in contracts they hope you'll just agree and not realize what you're signing, when in reality it would be better to negotiate something more reasonable and mutually beneficial. Do not assume businesses will do the right thing if you didn't realize what you were signing until later down the line.

Time Management, Negativity, and Theft

As you start to dive deeper into your business, you may find it difficult to manage your time between your day job and your blogging business. The same principles in which we as nurses are so accustomed to in our bedside world are applicable in a blogging business as well. Managing your time is critical, and successful prioritization and delegation are a must to grow your platform. We'll outline some good strategies and tips here, but we do recommend that you review the references section for additional resources on these and related topics.

Prioritization

Like the bedside, there are so many things that need to be done that it can be difficult to figure out which to address first. It is helpful to develop a strategy to address all of your needs, and then decide what is most important and will move the needle the farthest. Identify your tasks, and then categorize them into things that need to be done now, later, and someday. Think of the emergency department triage nurse who is seeing patients and deciding if the patient is emergent, urgent, or non-urgent. What needs to be done as soon as possible? What can wait a bit? And what can wait even longer? Thinking about tasks in this manner will help you not only be more productive, but also seem more productive to your audience.

For example, don't spend a week trying to figure out how to trademark your brand when you haven't come up with a new blog post in a month. That's kind of like the bedside nurse trying to restock all of the supply carts when his or her patient needs a new IV.

Organization is key, especially with so many moving pieces. Creating a calendar and schedule are really helpful. You may find it useful to create a blog editorial content calendar separate from your actual calendar of events, calls, and meetings. If you have an assistant, you can create a shared document (in Google Drive, for example) so they have access to a constantly updated calendar and know what's planned on being posted in the future.

Another method is to use a project or task management system. There are many free and paid tools available. Gqueues is a great tool if you use Google Chrome and Gmail because it integrates seamlessly. While there is a free version, the paid version is well worth the cost as it comes with several nice features. You can create several different task lists, recurring tasks, attach notes, documents, and due dates, and assign the task to someone else to complete. The tasks with due dates show up on your calendar. You can even turn emails into tasks. So rather than have an inbox overflowing with unread mail, you can create tasks based upon their urgency.

Create a schedule and stick to it. Your readers expect consistency. So, whether you're posting once a week or once a month, stick with it, down to the day, if at all possible. You can plan ahead and make this much more manageable. So, if life happens, your blog won't go dark.

If you put up a blog post once per week and it takes you a few hours to write one, you can set one full day aside for you to write your blog posts for the month, an afternoon to edit and format, and an evening to schedule and create feature images. By creating a set schedule to create your cornerstone pieces of content, you don't have to worry about scrambling to write a blog post the night before you want it posted.

Keep your ideas for content all in one place. There are so many things you could write about, but you may find it challenging if you haven't jotted down those great blog post ideas the moment you had them. You can take notes about potential topics in a notebook or your phone to reference when you actually sit down to write.

Creating a content calendar enables you to have more freedom with the rest of your time. You'll be able to have more time to engage with your audience on social. You won't have to worry about finding time to post links to your social media platforms because you know it's already scheduled. And don't forget to schedule time to un-plug.

Delegation

As your business and audience grows, so will your task list. If you're doing it right, so will your income. The more contracts, jobs, meetings, and so forth you take on, the less time you have for other things. This is similar to the bedside nurse who keeps getting admission after admission. Soon, it makes sense for you to focus on the tasks that only you as the nurse and business owner can do. This typically consists of just content including clinical knowledge and business strategy. Delegating tasks to others goes from being helpful to necessary. Start to think about the things that you don't have to do yourself. If possible, start with the thing you least enjoy.

Kati's Experience

It would typically take me about 1-1.5 hours to write a good blog post if I already had a topic in mind. However, I was noticing that it would take me another hour to format, tag, categorize, and look at SEO, and then another 1.5-2 hours to create an appealing image, and post a link to all of my social platforms. I was wasting a lot of time doing something that I could delegate/outsource. I hired an assistant and someone to create images for me. While technically I could do those tasks myself and it appeared to be cheaper, I found I was losing revenue. Those additional three hours spent formatting, editing, tagging, sharing, and so forth, could have been spent creating new content. As soon as I outsourced these tasks and could focus solely on content creation, my productivity skyrocketed.

As you're spending time creating videos, blog posts, social media shares, sending invoices, managing your books, reading contracts, and so forth, start to think about things you could potentially delegate.

So, who do you delegate to?

People tend to think that if they want hire someone to help with these things, it will be too expensive... Wrong! There are many freelancers who work for very reasonable rates. Many of the tasks necessary to maintain a blog can be delegated to a virtual assistant (VA).

VAs can do tasks like formatting blogs, scheduling social media, and maintaining a content calendar. Some will have additional skills and be able to create images or website design. If they don't possess a skill themselves, they can research and find a contractor to provide this service as they coordinate all the work.

It potentially will take them less time than if you did it, save you from headaches and the stress of researching how to do some of these things, and free you up to do what you do best: create content for your niche. Ultimately, it will cost you less to delegate than doing all the work yourself. If you earn $40 an hour as a nurse, and pay $10 an hour to your VA, he or she can do four times the amount of work for the same cost of as an hour of your time.

Brittney's Experience

Hiring a VA was one of the best decisions I ever made for my blog. I struggled with the idea of letting someone else into my bubble. I was worried they wouldn't post things correctly, that I would have to do things over again, or that they could potentially tarnish the reputation of my brand. However, I was at a transition period in my life and I didn't have the time to spend on blog tasks that I once did. My choice was clear: hire a VA or see the brand and business crumble.

When I took the plunge, I was so scared, but I spent a long time weeding through candidates, reading references, and finally found one that was a good fit for me.

My VA is a clone of me in many aspects of my business. She is so clear on the brand and message and can even speak in my voice. She does blog formatting, communicates with other brands, and organizes the content calendar. She also coordinates with other freelancers who produce images and other content for the site. I'd be lost without her.

As you grow and hire new contractors, you can develop a team. The more you can empower your team to function independently, the better. Thankfully, you're a nurse who is experienced in leading a healthcare team; leading your business team should be similar! Give your team specific directions, empower them to make decisions after they've proved they are capable, and provide encouragement and praise. The more who are excited to be on your team, the better. It will enable you to grow faster, earn more revenue, and help more people.

Your needs will change as your business grows. Some responsibilities that you may think about contracting out include:

- Virtual assistant
  - Blog editing
  - Content calendar
  - Social media
  - Checking email
- Bookkeeper - look for someone you trust who is experienced in the programs you want to utilize (QuickBooks, for example)
- Lawyer - look for someone who is experienced in reviewing contracts, copyright, trademarks, and intellectual property
- Accountant
- Graphic designer
- WordPress developer

Additionally, look into which tasks can be automated. Refer to the list of great social media apps and tools that can help you schedule your content provided in Chapter 8.

Boundaries

In the digital age in which we live, it is easy to slip into the "constantly accessible state." When you have your social media applications on your phone, notification turned on, and everyone with your personal cell number, it can be difficult to step away from your business. However, it is imperative to regularly have time off.

Kati's Experience

I originally made myself too accessible. I had my email address on my website, encouraging nurses or students who were struggling to contact me personally. I responded to messages as soon as they were received. I stayed up late answering non-urgent emails, compromising time with my loved ones. I found that people would just email me questions instead of looking at the mountains of resources I had created that already provided the answers.

I decided to step back. I took my email down and changed it to a contact form. I made sure the blog posts were categorized appropriately. If people reached out on social media, I'd have concise, yet genuine responses. I stopped obsessively checking my email. I directed the contact form to go to my assistant's email, and asked her to forward me anything that needed my attention specifically. My engagement continues to increase, as do business requests, but I have gained significant time back. Whenever I sit down to create, I'm not bogged down by all the emails and lapsed correspondence.

As the business owner, you want to be able to address needs as soon as possible. While the hospital never closes, you can turn your business off for a while to enjoy your life. In order to do this effectively, planning ahead is a must.

Therefore, be accessible to your audience through engagement on social media - on your timetable and terms. Make your content very easy to navigate so people don't feel the need to email you for every little question. Create avenues for people to contact you (like a contact form with specific drop down options related to the type of request). Empower your team (your assistant, your web designer) to function as independently as possible, so you can enjoy your business and downtime.

Why work 80 hours a week when you could work less than 20 and be just as productive, if not more? If you strive to be as effective possible, delegate and automate. Do not wear an 80-hour workweek like a badge of honor. Work hard on your business, but have boundaries. You truly need to be a little more proactive about this when you work from home. When you're working at the hospital or an office, you can just leave. But if you work from home, you're always at home/work and therefore need to exercise more restraint and boundaries when work time is done for the day or week.

If you're working 80 hours each week, just trying to get to the weekend, you're doing this wrong.

Negativity

Negativity online is quite rampant. The internet trolls are always hard at work trying to make as many people feel as miserable as they do. People say things online they would never say in person. They don't have to look the person in the eye and actually verbalize their hurtful commentary, can be passive-aggressive with little to no accountability, and don't get that immediate response from the person they are being negative to or about. Also, people can sometimes gang up on others easily because there is strength in numbers. Trolls can also hide within a sea of comments and not take accountability for their actions. Many times, it requires much less courage to type something that can reach thousands, than to have an honest one-on-one conversation with someone.

Do yourself a favor: Don't feed the trolls.

If you are growing an online business, you will eventually run into negativity. None of us are immune. Even if you are the nicest person in the world, someone will have a problem with you. In fact, sometimes this negatively is a clear indicator that you're successful.

Know this: You are not pizza. You can't please everyone.

There are a few important things to understand about negativity as a blogger.

First, people are easily offended. Even if you try to say something with the most grace possible, people still may respond poorly. This is especially the case if you post anything remotely resembling a political opinion or a polarizing topic.

Second, everyone is watching. Have you ever read something on social media where the original post wasn't too bad, but the comments got pretty ugly? Did you want to see how the original poster responded? And did you comment? Arguably, most people watch these things unfold online and very few chime into the conversation. For people to jump into the conversation, they typically have to get pretty heated. People watch closely how bloggers, business owners, etc. respond to negativity about them or their brand online. Therefore, be careful how you respond.

Finally, try to take the emotion out of it. Or rather, use your emotional intelligence to channel your feelings appropriately. Step away from it for a while and then approach the negative person online like you would if you had a patient or loved one speak to you in that manner. Try to read what they've said objectively and not have an emotion-filled response. If reading it makes you angry, step back. Process the situation with someone whose judgment you trust (ideally, your accountability partner we discussed earlier in the book) and try to let that initial gut response calm down before diving in. If a response is necessary, provide an appropriate one. Rarely are these issues squashed with one response. Typically, the negative person will again respond and you must choose if you want to continue to engage or not.

Kati's Brush with Negativity

I regularly post live videos on Facebook. Facebook Live has a comment feature. I once did a demo of a basic assessment of a neurologically compromised patient in a neurointensive care unit. While most comments were overwhelmingly positive, there were two that were quite negative. One woman said, "Wow, that's how you would assess a stroke patient? Major fail." And another woman said, "OMG why is she talking so much?!" I didn't see the comments until I was done with the demo and going through the comments one-by-one to make sure I answered the questions. I was a bit caught off guard, hurt, and also bummed to hear those kinds of comments when I was taking time out of my day to provide that demo, but responded to both in a respectful, yet firm way. I knew if I flew off the handle, I would just look like I couldn't control myself. I also knew hundreds of people were watching how I would respond. Actually, multiple other viewers responded to their comments before I even saw them, and thanked me for my time. When I went back to review the video the next day to see if anyone had any additional comments, those two women had deleted their original comments.

Brittney's Negative Learning Experience

I've received several critiques of my grammar over the years. Some of them were hateful, public comments challenging my intelligence and ability to care for patients. When you write online this is going to happen. I grew very frustrated by this initially, but I actually used this as an opportunity to improve. I became more aware of my need to pay attention to potential grammatical errors. I also invest in additional tools to check my grammar automatically. Ultimately, I decided that having a VA review my content was a good use of resources and no longer encounter this particular version of negativity.

Not all negativity deserves or requires a response. If it's incredibly inappropriate, you may want to just think about deleting the comment (which goes back to our point on creating a comment policy!), especially if it's explicit. Remember, this is your blog, your social media, and your space. You don't *have* to have anything on there you don't want, or anything that makes you uncomfortable. You wouldn't let someone come in your house and destroy your beautiful hardwoods, don't let them do it online.

Theft

When you create amazing content, people will become inspired by and want to imitate you. You may eventually find that rather than using your content as inspiration, someone has actually placed your content in full on their website. If you've noticed this has happened, remain calm. It's easy to get heated about this immediately when someone has stolen from you, especially if it's something that meant a great deal to you. First, try to contact them directly with a firm, but kind email (or contact form) requesting them to remove your content or provide appropriate attribution.

If you do not receive a response or your work has not been removed, you can contact their host and file a DMCA takedown request. This will force the site to remove the content or risk their entire site being taken offline until they do so.

If this does not resolve the issue, consider discussing the matter with your lawyer. They may advise issuing a cease and desist order. This is kind of like when you're trying to calm your agitated patient, you don't just jump straight for the four-point restraints... the same is true here. Use the least amount of intervention, if possible. A firm no and redirection will hopefully do the trick, but if not, this still leaves you quite a bit of room to escalate if needed.

Brittney's Experience

I've had many instances where people copy entire blog posts and paste on their own sites. Several of these have been travel and staffing companies. Usually I contact and politely explain that my work is copyright and have not authorized them to republish my content. Usually they did not realize what they did was wrong, and correct the mistake by removing my content and profusely apologizing.

I did have one site (a training company) that copied several pieces of my content and refused to respond to any of my attempts to communicate with them. Because of their lack of response, I was forced to resort to filing a DMCA takedown request with their host. They also neglected to respond to the DMCA within the specified time frame and their entire site was taken down. It wasn't my intent to harm their business, but they were harming mine by stealing my content.

Therefore, make sure you're monitoring your brand and business. Look at your competitors' websites and social media once in a while and see what people are saying about you. Search your name and brand on various social media platforms and see what people are saying. Set up Google Alerts with your name and your blog/brand name. You won't know if people are stealing from you or speaking negatively about you if you don't look around. It's helpful to know the image your brand has in the social space online, and being clued into this will enable you to find out if your content has been stolen, and if you creating a good reputation within your niche.

CHAPTER 10

PUTTING IT ALL
TOGETHER

Take a deep breath, you're almost done.
Ok. That's not true. Building a brand online is never really done.
However, you have made it through nine action-packed chapters. That's something to celebrate. Keep the cork on the bottle for a few more minutes; we need to put a bow on this package.

In Chapter 1 we focused on the power and potential of blogging. You can use a blog to grow and develop both personally and professionally. Nurses have a unique skillset which makes them great bloggers and business owners. You can combine your passions in patient care with the nearly limitless reach of the internet to positively impact the nursing profession and your own professional and personal goals.

We covered defining your message and niche in Chapter 2. Before you really jump in feet first, it's important to clearly define your focus including your bottom line and your specific niche. The more specific you can get, the better. Your online presence and the overall brand and image you put out in the world will be the foundation of your business. Getting an accountability partner at this stage in the game can really help you keep your momentum going to reach your long-term business goals.

Chapter 3 focused on branding and consistency. We walked you through determining whether your blog should be a personal brand or have more of a business presence. There are certainly pros and cons of each, and there is no right or wrong decision. Once you've made that decision you'll decide on a name and tagline. That choice will then help form your logo and may even impact the color and font choices that will ultimately make up your branding kit. Yes, branding kit. You need one of those. It just makes things easier in the long run. Trust us.

The nerdy fun started in Chapter 4. We outlined the steps to start a blog including the information you need to know on hosting, domain names, plugins, posts, pages, and much more. This chapter is packed with resources, definitions, and explanations for some of the most common technical questions faced when developing a blog.

Even if you see the value, your brand is on point, and you've got all the technical stuff in place, you won't be doing anyone any favors without amazing content. Chapter 5 was all about ensuring each post is awesome. We walked you through some of the most common mistakes and provided recommended practices so you can avoid many of the costly and frustrating blogger pitfalls.

Your content has no value if it is not seen. Chapter 6 is all about how to ensure that people actually read your blog. We outline key principles around SEO, email lists, and social media that will drive traffic when used effectively.

This blogging stuff is super easy and no one would ever expect to earn any money from it. Not. Pardon us for channeling our inner Wayne Campbell, but it just had to be done. Seriously, though, Chapter 7 was all about income streams, both active and passive. There are so many ways you can use a blog to earn income and we've included some of the most popular and effective.

Part of building a blog is ensuring that you've also built a complimenting social media presence. In Chapter 8 we dissect each social network and discuss how to reach each audience effectively. Remember, you can't just copy and paste the same 140 character message across all your channels. Each network fulfills a distinct purpose and content must be crafted specifically for that audience's needs.

Chapter 9 fills in some gaps around practical details. From legal considerations to prioritization and delegation, this chapter is your resource for keeping your sanity and your livelihood in the long run.

If you gain nothing else from this chapter, utilize the time manage and delegation principles including hiring a V.A. Do it as soon as you can afford it.

That brings us to this chapter. Chapter 10, the final chapter is here to wrap everything up and put a nice big bow on it. It's a decompress chapter, that's also relatively short. In fact, you've only got a handful of paragraphs left. Whew.

We'll round out this book by describing your blogging business utilizing more HGTV references than you might anticipate. (Hint: 1) Stay with us, you're almost done.

Building a Blog Home

Defining your passion and bottom line is the foundation of your business home. If your foundation isn't sturdy and truly important to you, then it will not stand the test of time or be able to weather the storms. Build your house on stone, not sand.

Your accountability partner is your watchful eye, who lets you know if shingles are falling down, the roof needs to be replaced, or if someone has broken a window. They can also help to keep you on track when you set goals. Please do not underestimate the power of trustful outside eyes and a firm, but reassuring, voice.

Once you have your foundation solid, then you can start to design the exterior of your home: your brand identity. It is essential that the identity is cohesive and simply makes sense. You don't want bricks on one side, siding on another, and shiplap on another (even if that would make Joanna Gaines happy). Your blog is not a fixer upper. Your blog is your business. A consistent and clear brand is a must.

Then, it's time to really jump in and do the dirty work: the structure. Your website and social media platforms all must be set up appropriately to make sure everything runs smoothly, it's easy to navigate, and remains supported.

While the inter-workings of your blog are the internal structure of your home, your content is your floors, drywall, fixtures, furniture, and appliances. You don't want your home to have bare drywall, a stove from 1958, no lighting, a couch found off the street, and an air mattress in your master bedroom. No. You want stainless steel appliances, high-quality interior paint, recessed can lighting, a comfortable and clean couch, and a four-post king-sized master bed with a duvet so puffy you could get lost in it.

You can have the best internal structure ever, but if you don't have a comfortable and enjoyable interior, no one is going to stay long. They're going to run inside, get what they need from you and exit faster than a nurse clocking out after their shift.

You must put time, love, and care into creating an enjoyable interior/quality content that speaks directly to your audience.

But creating this wonderful atmosphere and home is all in vain if you can't turn the lights on. You must be able to afford to keep it running, which is why monetization is absolutely key.

Your house isn't a home unless it has touches of you throughout it, which is where social media comes in. Maybe you appreciate history and like historical touches, maybe you are more sleek and modern, or maybe you're humorous and laid back. People get to know you through social media, so make sure your personality is evident.

And finally, your roof is the practical considerations we discussed: forming a corporation, tax considerations, contracts, legal aspects and so forth. Ideally, these are things you put in place early on and it will keep you safe for years to come, much like a quality roof. Buying a new roof for a home is not just a worthwhile investment, but also a necessary one. All of your beautiful walls, floors, and even your puffy duvet could come crashing down without a proper roof. (Not the duvet!)

Build your blog to the best of your ability with the knowledge you have, but also knowing that you'll always be able to update things later. Just like in nursing, a blogger never stops learning. The rules change, recommended practices evolve, and new social media channels are constantly emerging. Your single biggest asset as a professional blogger will be your ability to adapt and evolve with the changing needs of the digital world.

You can do it. We have faith in you. You are a nurse after all! If you can bring someone back to life, you can certainly blog.

The End is Only the Beginning

But now the end is near, and we must face the final challenge of wrapping up this book.

We hope you have enjoyed this information, and that it will help you build your business.

Thank you for not only being a nurse - which is a thank you that could span an entire book - but thank you for being so engaged within our profession that you want to take it to the next level with creating your own blog and business.

This may be the end of this book, but it's only the beginning of the next phase of your blogging journey.

References

View references including urls at HealthMediaAcademy.com/ references

An, Mimi. "Average Traffic Sources For Websites: Benchmarks From 15K HubSpot Customers". *Research.hubspot.com*. N.p., 2016. Web. 24 Mar. 2017.

Aslam, Salmon. "Pinterest By The Numbers (2017): Stats, Demographics & Fun Facts".

Barry, Chris. "Putting Social Media To Work". Bain.com. N.p., 2011. Web. 24 Mar. 2017

Brinker, Mark. "7 Little-Known Reasons Wordpress.Com Sucks For Serious Bloggers • Smart Blogger". *Smart Blogger*, 2017, https:// smartblogger.com/wordpress-hosting/.

Chaffey, Dave. "Email Marketing Statistics 2016 Compilation". *Smart Insights*. N.p., 2016. Web. 24 Mar. 2017.

Clark, Alexander. "Search Engine Statistics". *Smart Insights*. N.p., 2017. Web. 23 Mar. 2017

"Contact Form 7". *WordPress.org*. N.p., 2017. Web. 23 Mar. 2017.

Dean, Brian. "We Analyzed 1 Million Google Search Results. Here's What We Learned About SEO". *Backlinko*. N.p., 2016. Web. 24 Mar. 2017.

DeMers, Jayson. "Social Media Now Drives 31% Of All Referral Traffic". *Forbes.com*. N.p., 2015. Web. 23 Mar. 2017.

"Facebook Remains The Most Popular Social Media Platform". *Pew Research Center: Internet, Science & Tech*. N.p., 2016. Web. 25 Mar. 2017.

"The FTC'S Endorsement Guides: What People Are Asking | Federal Trade Commission". *Ftc.gov*. N.p., 2017. Web. 23 Mar. 2017.

Hyatt, Michael S. Platform: Get Noticed In A Noisy World. 1st ed. Nashville, Tenn.: Thomas Nelson, 2012. Print.

K, Karol. "The Ultimate List Of WordPress Statistics". *CodeinWP Blog*. N.p., 2017. Web. 23 Mar. 2017.

Kirkpatrick, David. "Most Of Facebook's 8B Daily Video Views Happen Without Sound". *Marketing Dive*. N.p., 2016. Web. 25 Mar. 2017

Krook, Nienke. "How To Write A Disclaimer For Your Blog | The Travel Tester". *The Travel Tester*. N.p., 2012. Web. 23 Mar. 2017.

"Nursing Statistics | Minority Nurse". *Minoritynurse.com*. N.p., 2013. Web. 25 Mar. 2017.

Omnicoreagency.com. N.p., 2017. Web. 25 Mar. 2017

Schwartz, Eli. "Is Google's Search Market Share Actually Dropping?". *Search Engine Land*. N.p., 2015. Web. 23 Mar. 2017.

Sharp, Eric. "The First Page Of Google, By The Numbers". Protofuse.com. N.p., 2014. Web. 23 Mar. 2017

"Shopping Stats: People Pin In A Buying State-Of-Mind". *for Business*. N.p., 2015. Web. 25 Mar. 2017.

"Terms Of Service". *Wordpress.Com*, 2017, http://en.wordpress.com/tos.

The Ultimate List Of Blog Post Ideas". *DigitalMarketer*. N.p., 2015. Web. 23 Mar. 2017.

Vaynerchuk, Gary. *Jab, Jab, Jab, Right Hook: How to Tell Your Story in a Noisy, Social World*. First edition. HarperBusiness, 2013.

Walters, Kendall. "The Facebook Algorithm: What You Need To Know To Boost Organic Reach". *Hootsuite Social Media Management*. N.p., 2016. Web. 25 Mar. 2017

"What Do Over 80% Of Employers Do BEFORE Inviting You To An Interview? | CHE Career Exploration Center". *Blogs.cornell.edu.* N.p., 2014. Web. 25 Mar. 2017.

"What Is A DMCA Takedown? - DMCA.Com". *DMCA Protection & Takedown Services,* 2017, https://www.dmca.com/FAQ/What-is-a-DMCA-Takedown.

Wong, Danny. "Report: Social Media Drove 31.24% Of Overall Visits To Sites". *The Shareaholic Content Marketing Blog.* N.p., 2017. Web. 23 Mar. 2017.

Appendix A:
Definitions

Affiliate Marketing: A mechanism to earn income online by promotion relevant products or services with special tracking links. Each purchase earns a commission.

Aggregator: A service that groups related content, programs, or tools in a single location.

Analytics: Systematic analysis of data. Specifically, Google Analytics provides analysis of data related to website visits.

Backlinks: A link back to your website from an external source. These links may be dofollow or nofollow, depending on the source of the link. For example, social sites generally give nofollow links while guest blogging generally nets dofollow links.

Brand Ambassador: A person that is paid in exchange or endorsement or mentions of a product or service.

Branding: An identity, tone, or feel related to a product, service, company, or individual.

Categories: A portion of the taxonomy used to sort and categorize content into related groups. Related to broad topics. Like chapters of a book.

Clickbait: Is a post where the title or copy try to get someone to click on a link, out of curiosity, but won't end up providing value.

Click Through Rate: Describes the percentage of subscribers that click on a link within the body of an email. The higher the better.

CMS: Content management system. A program that manages content and automatically creates links and connections when new content is added.

Content: A broad term describing text, images, video, and other media used in creation of a blog and related promotion.

CPC: Cost per click. Advertisers pay every time an ad is clicked.

CPM: Cost per million impressions. Advertisers pay per 1,000 ad views.

CSS: Cascading Style Sheets is a markup language that deals with the style and representation of your website. CSS impacts your fonts, to colors, to size and locations of tables and DIVs, CSS is what you'll adjust.

Curated: Content that is carefully selected and edited for optimal presentation

cPanel: A control panel that includes automation tools, software installation, and settings for websites.

Dashboard: The administrative panel or backend of WordPress. The location where you update content, adjust theme and style, manage plugins, and other administrative functions.

Database: A system of related tables. In blog terms, a database is the structure that holds all text data on a blog. This includes all words written in a post. It is what makes the CMS of WordPress function.

DMCA Takedown: "When content is removed from a website at the request of the owner of the content or the owner of the copyright of the content;8" and DMCA stands for The Digital Millennium Copyright Act. (https://www.dmca.com/FAQ/What-is-a-DMCA-Takedown)

Dofollow: An attribute assigned to a URL that tells Google and other search engines that the link can, and should, be used to influence search results. This is the default, and typically not needed, but may be the case if you have installed a plugin that makes all external links nofollow. This is accomplished by adding rel="dofollow". Example: <a href="http://www.google.com/" rel="dofollow">Google</a>

Endorsement: A recommendation of a product or service. Payment may or may not have changed hands.

Freelance Writing: Writing that is paid either per-word, per page, or a flat fee.

Headings: A mechanism for breaking up and grouping related content in a post or page.

H1: Heading 1. This will be your title and WordPress will create this automatically. Do not create an H1 within the content of your post.

H2: Heading 2. This will be the main themes of your post. These break up content and describe the content found within.

H3: Heading 3. This will further break up content in an H2 in lengthy posts or where it makes sense to further divide content.

Health Insurance Portability and Accountability Act (HIPAA): Is a privacy standard for healthcare professionals that ensures that information about a specific patient or encounter is on a need to know basis. If confidentiality is breached, fines and other penalties will apply.

Hosting: The act of hosting a website.

Javascript: Computer language that creates actions on an object on a webpage. Often these actions occur on click.

Keyword: The word or phrase your content is about. Ideally your keywords are highly searched with low competition.

Monetize: To earn revenue from

Niche: A small specialized topic or focus that appeals to a small subset of the population.

Nofollow: An attribute you can assign to a URL to tell Google and other search engines to not count this link when determining search ranking. In short, it makes sure your link doesn't impact where that page appears in Google search results. This is accomplished by adding rel="nofollow". Example: <a href="http://www.google.com/" rel="nofollow">Google</a>

One-off: A single instance. One-off deals, posts, or work is usually a single blog post or a set number of social media shares without the expectation of long term or recurring work.

Opt-in: The act of agreeing to be included. An opt-in can also reference a free resource provided in exchange for someone giving you their email and agreeing to receive email notifications.

Organic: Content that is raw, unedited, and typically unsolicited. Also, content that is written without payment or appears in search results without payment.

Page: A type of content on a blog that contains content that is typically more static in nature. Often for resources and routinely linked items.

Page Rank (SERP): How high a specific page or post will appear when someone Google's a certain term. The higher the better.

Passive Income Stream: An income stream that will consistently pay out with little or no added work. Rental properties are a great example.

Plugin: A add-on to functionality of WordPress enabling new features. Paid and free available. Like apps for WordPress.

Post: A type of content on a blog that is created routinely. These are the main components of a blog.

Search Engine Optimization (SEO): The art of and science of writing content in such a way that search engines rank your content higher in SERP, and readers find your highly valuable content when looking to solve their specific problem, related to your keywords.

Search Engine Results Page (SERP): Used interchangeably with page rank. This is the ranking a specific page has for a specific search term.

SoMe: Social Media. Websites and services that allow you to connect and share information with friends, family, peers, or others.

Sponsored Posts: Blog posts that have been paid for in either money, products, or service.

Sponsorship: Generally relating to a financial relationship in which a blog or influencer is paid for specific groups of services for a set period of time. A sponsorship can extend beyond a blog into social media channels.

Table: Content displayed in columns. Also refers to the underlying architecture of a WordPress Database.

Tags: A portion of the taxonomy used to sort and categorize content into related groups. Related to narrow topics. Like terms in an index.

Theme: The look and feel of a blog. Can be installed pre-made or made custom.

VA: Virtual Assistant. An online assistant that can complete tasks as assigned. The type of tasks depends of the skillset of the assistant.

Widget: A block of content generated by code either from an integrated or connected service. Many are built in with WordPress. Others can be added by plugin.

WordPress: A popular and free content management system for blogs and websites.

Appendix B:
Recommended Resources

Please visit HealthMediaAcademy.com/resources for a full list of every resource mentioned throughout this book, as well as a few more! We list books, applications, programs, plugins, and more. We link directly to them all so that you know it is exactly what you're looking for.

Made in the USA
Columbia, SC
23 June 2019